Psychology Revivals

Brain, Mind, and the External Signs of Intelligence

Born in Vienna in 1864, Bernard Hollander was a London-based psychiatrist in the early twentieth century. He is best known for being one of the main proponents of the interest in phrenology at that time. This title originally published in 1931 looks at the different regions of the brain and their various functions in relation to intelligence. From the preface: "The records of cases collected by the author, including some of his own, point to there being at least three main regions of totally different functions.... Of these three regions, the frontal is by far the largest in man and the most important, being the region for the manifestation of the highest intellectual abilities." Back in print this is a chance to read all about the study of the brain, mind and external signs of intelligence from the early twentieth century.

Brain, Mind, and the External Signs of Intelligence

Bernard Hollander

Routledge
Taylor & Francis Group
LONDON AND NEW YORK

First published in 1931
by George Allen & Unwin Ltd

This edition first published in 2015 by Routledge
27 Church Road, Hove BN3 2FA

and by Routledge
711 Third Avenue, New York, NY 10017

Routledge is an imprint of the Taylor & Francis Group, an informa business

Publisher's Note
The publisher has gone to great lengths to ensure the quality of this reprint but points out that some imperfections in the original copies may be apparent.

Disclaimer
The publisher has made every effort to trace copyright holders and welcomes correspondence from those they have been unable to contact.

A Library of Congress record exists under LCCN: 32007493

ISBN: 978-1-138-84153-6 (hbk)
ISBN: 978-1-315-73211-4 (ebk)

BRAIN, MIND, AND THE EXTERNAL SIGNS OF INTELLIGENCE

by

BERNARD HOLLANDER, M.D.

Corresponding Member of The Royal Academy of Medicine of Madrid

ILLUSTRATED

LONDON

GEORGE ALLEN & UNWIN LTD

MUSEUM STREET

FIRST PUBLISHED IN 1931

PRINTED IN GREAT BRITAIN BY
UNWIN BROTHERS LTD., WOKING

PREFACE

Of all the organs in the human body, the brain is of the greatest interest, and ranks highest in importance; yet a survey of the views of the recognised authorities of the present day, as given in this book, tends to show that, whereas other branches of medical science have made great advances during the past hundred years, the physiology of the brain presents such difficulties that our knowledge of the *mental* functions is still obscure.

One of the reasons for this lack of progress is that brain research has hitherto been hampered by psychological dogmas almost as effectively as it was by theological dogmas in earlier times.

Consequently, we have not got beyond the vague statement that the brain is *the organ of the mind*, and there is no agreement as to what is meant by the term "mind", or what is its relation to the brain.

It is only a little more than a century since the search for the seat of the "soul" in the brain has been given up; and only about sixty years since the brain has ceased to be regarded as a uniform organ, on the ground of the unity of the "ego" and the indivisibility of the mind.

Even to-day many investigators still regard mind as if it consisted exclusively of the lofty intellect of man, and completely ignore the emotions and instinctive dispositions for the preservation of self and the species, which also are part of the mind, and which indeed in animals form almost the entire mind—their intellect being only rudimentary.

Sixty years ago it was confidently anticipated that experiments on the exposed brains of living animals would speedily disclose the nature of the mind and the inner working of the brain, and make mental disorders disappear for ever. But, as is well known, these extravagant hopes have not been fulfilled.

All that experimental physiology succeeded in doing was to localise centres in the brain, where sensations are received and the response is given to muscular movements; but the mind, which makes use of these centres, has, so far, escaped discovery.

It is now realised that neither electrical stimulation nor the destruction of portions of an animal's brain—which were the two accepted methods of investigation—could ever shed light on the diversity of human talents and dispositions, or the variety of mental derangements.

It has been found, moreover, that the sensory and motor centres, that had been successfully localised, are not—as was originally believed—cortical, i.e. on the surface of the brain, but subcortical. For the paralysis which ensues upon the destruction of their respective areas—whether done experimentally or following accident or disease—is only temporary. It is not surprising, therefore, that this method of research has now been given up.

In consequence of these failures, many experts have reverted to the old view of a century ago, which regarded the brain as being a uniform organ, and localisation of function therefore impossible.

Great results were also expected from the study of the microscopical anatomy of the cortex of the brain; but, though we have learnt much about the configuration of the various layers of brain cells, and their arrangement in structurally differentiated territories, there still prevail conflicting opinions as to the significance of these discoveries.

The fact is that neither thought nor feeling can be lifted

with the scalpel; nor will a brain section held under the magnifying lens reveal its living function.

Instances will be quoted of the brains of men of renown having been cut into as many as thirty thousand minute sections, a wonderful feat in itself; yet we have learnt very little from it, not knowing what signs to look for as indicating individual greatness.

Notwithstanding a vast amount of research, nothing is known why one man's genius should take the direction of a Newton, while that of another develops into a Shakespeare or a Michel Angelo. Nothing is known to explain why one man should become saintly in character, while another develops into a genius of crime.

But, because the investigations hitherto pursued have proved unsatisfactory, this is no reason why we should rest content with our present knowledge or lack of knowledge; for there may be other methods more fruitful of results.

Now that experiments on animals have apparently reached their limit of usefulness, a more promising method for advancing our knowledge of the mental functions of the brain would be the collection of clinical and pathological data, such as are given with abundant detail in this book: by observing the effects of cerebral injury and circumscribed disease on man; since he alone can communicate his feelings, sensations, and thoughts, by means of speech.

Usually, in such circumscribed lesions, one or more mental powers become deranged, while in other respects the individual remains perfectly sound; and, whenever the injury or disease affects the same locality, the same mental power suffers.

The records of cases collected by the author, including some of his own, point to there being at least three main regions of totally different functions: the frontal, parieto-occipital, and lower temporo-sphenoidal. Of these three regions, the frontal is by far the largest in man and the most important, being the region for the manifestation of the highest intellectual abilities.

Indeed, the evidence shows that, just as there are specific types of genius, so there are specific types of frontal brain: for mechanical science, philosophy, poetry, mathematics, music, and so forth.

Of course, not every man possessing such a type of brain will necessarily manifest that particular capacity. The gift alone is not enough. Among other conditions, he may lack the training, or may not possess the character qualities which urge men to work hard for the acquisition of knowledge.

The development of the frontal lobes, as the illustrations show, may be estimated in the living head. True, until recent years it was believed that the size and shape of the skull had no relation to the size and shape of the brain. Now, however, there is not an anatomist in existence who would deny that, for all practical purposes, skull and brain conform in outline.

But, if this is so, then it is highly desirable, without committing anyone to the tenets of any particular doctrine, that more attention be paid to the shape of the head.

We have expert histologists and pathologists—that is to say, experts of the post-mortem appearances of the brain—and even experts of prehistoric skulls; but, so far, the living head has had so little interest for medical men, that one would expect that the organ of the mind might be anywhere but in the cavity of the cranium.

Indeed, no one seems to know, nor has it ever been

scientifically explained, what is a good or a bad head; or what are the signs which indicate special intellectual abilities or definite character dispositions.

It was by the observation of living heads that the author discovered thirty years ago, among other important facts mentioned in this book, that a large number of feeble-minded children, though of normal parentage, were mentally deficient in consequence of injuries to their brain at birth, as the result of difficult labour, having malformed heads or bearing the marks of a badly applied forceps.

It is only within the last ten years that this has been more commonly recognised. Systematic investigation at Institutions for the Feeble-minded has revealed that 10 per cent. of the inmates were the victims of such injuries, and the evidence of brain surgeons will be quoted that if such lesions were attended to shortly after birth, subsequent mental and moral deficiency might be prevented.

However, it is not on cranioscopy, but on clinical evidence that the author bases his deductions. Such clinical observations have never been made systematically. The cases recorded in medical journals are so few that it requires a survey of the world's literature in order to obtain sufficient material; the paucity of reports being due, principally, to the common belief that localisation of *mental* functions in the brain is not possible.

Consequently—as will be shown by many examples quoted in this book—no definite psychological examination of the patient is made; and, often, the locality of the lesion is but vaguely described. It is not surprising, therefore, that destruction of large areas of the brain is sometimes recorded "without any mental change".

The evidence which will be given is not that of isolated

instances, but of hundreds of cases, incontrovertible in fact —including many which have been treated surgically with marked success.

These cases have not been chosen merely because they support the author's theories. Adverse facts and cases have been reported with equal fidelity.

Possibly some of the examples are not as perfect as can be desired; but they are the average that can be found in the world's medical literature.

Nor does the author claim, as some critics have stated, that all insane can be cured by surgical operation. Insanity is due to a variety of causes; sometimes it is of bodily origin. The operable cases refer only to head injury, circumscribed inflammation or haemorrhage, and brain tumours.

Altogether, it is not the author's wish that anything contained in this book should be taken for granted. It was written solely for the purpose of giving an impetus to a general inquiry into the whole problem of brain functions, on new lines. Research is needed: research by new methods, unhampered by dogma or false preconceptions.

For this purpose it is necessary that the future investigator should be acquainted with the failures of the past, in order to avoid repetition of the same errors; to this end, the historical and critical account of the chief theories and actual investigations should be of help, even to those who do not agree with the author's conclusions.

Unfortunately, such a history cannot be written—as, indeed, no new or partially known truth can be advocated—without opposing some "authority" or proving the failure of some branch of science, even when based on experiment or on the application of a recognised method of research.

Still, considering the present confusion with reference

to the most elementary problems of brain functions, such independent inquiry—though it has some faults and is opposed to current views—should not suffer the usual fate of being ignored, or treated off-handedly, if we have the advancement of knowledge genuinely at heart.

Anyone who has studied the history of medicine will know that medical opinions despised by one generation have often become the dogma of a later one.

Every attempt should be made to solve this problem of the functions of the brain. If this were done, on the lines adopted by the author in this work, new light would be shed on the whole subject of mental disorders—and on other disturbances of the brain, such as epilepsy, which the evidence shows to be most frequent in lesions of the temporal lobes.

The author, speaking with the knowledge derived from a lifelong study of the subject, feels convinced that the treatment of insanity will not be perfect until proper research has disclosed the localisation of the mental functions of the brain, and that such knowledge can hardly fail also to lead to the elucidation of some of the most difficult and interesting psychological, educational, and social problems.

Psychologists, if they wish to arrive at a real "science of mind", or to found a real "science of character"; teachers who want to draw out and make the most of the native abilities of the young; even social reformers anxious for the reduction of poverty, misconduct, vice, and crime—should possess an elementary knowledge of the brain and its functions, i.e. of the organic basis of the instincts, emotions, and higher mental attributes, in order to know what is innate in man and what is acquired, and to be able to distinguish the mentally deficient from the normal and those gifted in special directions.

Indeed, every man should know something of the brain mechanism with which he is endowed, to enable him to make the best use of it.

57 Wimpole Street
London, W. 1
1931

(*See also* Postscript, page 274)

CONTENTS

ILLUSTRATIONS

BRAIN, MIND, AND THE EXTERNAL SIGNS OF INTELLIGENCE

CHAPTER I

INTRODUCTION

The Nature of the Mind

The mind of man has been a subject of investigation and discussion for thousands of years; but, even to-day, we know very little of its nature. Though commonly spoken of as if it were an entity, mind as such is unknown. All that we actually know is *mental activities*, and the total of these we may, for convenience' sake, call mind.

Psychologists, until quite recent years, have concerned themselves greatly with the reason of man, as though the human mind comprised within its domain nothing further than mere intellect, but we all have instinctive dispositions which give rise to desires, and we all feel and strive as well as think. Even William James, the great philosopher, who furnished us with a new theory of emotions, devoted nine-tenths of his treatise on Psychology to the consideration of the Intellect, and only one-tenth to Feeling and Will.

To the metaphysicians of old, thought was all important; but thought is a secondary phenomenon, and arises only where spontaneous or reflex action is no longer active. If the animal is prompted by only one instinctive desire, it will act on impulse, that is, without hesitation, meditation, or reflection. But where several instincts are aroused at the same time—as when the animal at the sight of danger has the option of self-defence, running away, or hiding itself—there will be a delay in the response, giving rise to reflection and volition.

Animal instinct concerns itself only with the preservation of life and the means of living, and what intellect animals possess is employed toward that end. The mind of man is of far higher quality. It is not confined to a mere making provision for the flesh, as is the case with animals, but reaches far beyond this to something intellectual and spiritual; to things ethical and aesthetical. Man can rise intellectually to unknown heights because of his faculty of speech, which enables him to think in the abstract and gives him power of imagination; but he is moved by the same primitive impulses as the lower animals.

This observation can be confirmed by a study of the feeble-minded, in whom intellect is deficient, but the animal dispositions persist, often stronger from lack of control. This observation is further confirmed by a study of the infant mind, the instinctive dispositions of which are manifested long before the growth of the intellect. Indeed, our early education consists largely in curbing the animal desires or directing them into proper channels.

There is much controversy in regard to the instincts in man and their actual number, which has been stated by various writers to be as high as seventy and as low as three or four. When we are better acquainted with the mental functions of the brain, only such instincts will be admitted as primary which can be traced to definite regions of the brain, for all primary instincts depend upon a hereditary disposition of the nervous system.

When an instinct is aroused, it may result in spontaneous action. But if the action is delayed, the energy which would have gone to its realisation may be turned inward and give rise to certain feelings which move the entire organism, and because of that power to move, such feelings are called "emotions". Thus, the emotion of fear is aroused by the sight of danger, and the emotion of anger by the sight of opposition, or obstacles, or of an enemy.

Both emotions and instincts are forces within us which serve for the performance of certain functions. Both are inherited, and in nowise guided by conscious experience; though experience tends to modify, at least, the instincts, which then remain, more or less, as dispositions—a reason why the term "propensities" is sometimes applied to them. As all primary instincts tend to produce some form of emotional excitement, emotions have been described as the affective, or feeling, part of the instinct.

Propensities, whether in man or animals, give rise to desires for a particular end, but leave it almost entirely to reason to discover the means of attaining that end. If man were provided with instincts, and not merely propensities, he would not require such a long period of protection and instruction.

The greater the intellect of a man, the greater, as a rule, the check upon his emotions and passions. The lower the power of the intellect, the more freely do the feelings influence the actions of the individual. Therefore, a child, a savage, and persons of no culture, are little able to restrain their inclinations. This is the reason also why, in injuries to the intellectual region of the brain, there is so often loss of control over the propensities.

The intellectual capacities and the emotions are two distinct sets of mental powers; but, in their manifestation, are commonly blended together. A feeling of some kind arises at or about the same time as the idea, and is associated with it. On the other hand, just as the intellect may work independently, so the emotions may manifest themselves primarily without any ideas.

For example, there is often anxious feeling without any idea. The individual experiencing that feeling may seek for a cause, and may fasten upon some idea; but the feeling comes first. A man may be in a state of irritability, amounting to anger, before he has been opposed, or had occasion to find fault. It relieves him when he can discharge his anger on some individual or object, though he or it may be innocent of any offence.

Thoughts come and go; emotions last some time. When, for example, the emotion of fear is aroused, it may continue even when danger is passed. The emotions are not only far more extensive in their action than the intellect, but are more important for health and sanity. In mental derangement, the primary disorder usually consists in a tendency to disordered emotion, which affects the course of thought, and, consequently, of action, without disordering the reasoning processes in any other way than by supplying them with wrong materials.

To understand emotional action, it is necessary to take note of the fact that we have, besides the nerves of the five senses, two systems of nerves: (1) the voluntary, or cerebrospinal, and (2) the involuntary, or sympathetic. The *cerebrospinal system* originates in the brain, and runs inside the spinal column in the hollow of the vertebrae. It consists of nerves of sensation, which carry messages from the surface of the body to the brain; and of nerves of motion, which, in response to the sensations, carry out muscular movements. The *sympathetic system* is situated within the body, along each side of the spinal column, and consists of a number of collections of nerve matter—so-called ganglia—from which

Plate I

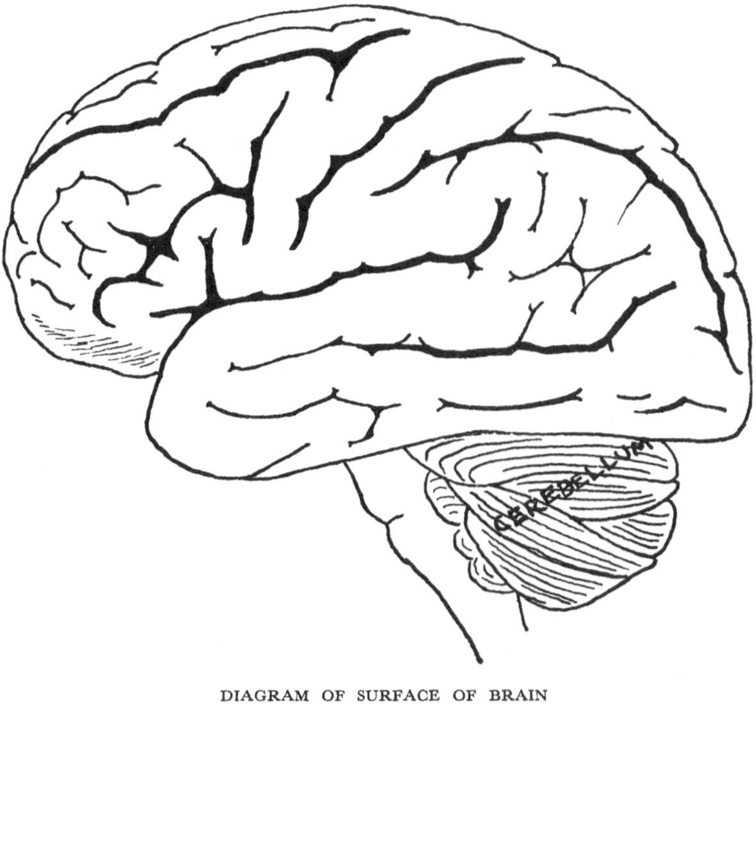

DIAGRAM OF SURFACE OF BRAIN

branch off fine networks of nerve fibres which go to all the internal organs, as well as to the blood vessels, glands, and to the cerebro-spinal nerves, helping to increase or check muscular movement.

When the response to an external stimulus is effected through the voluntary, or cerebro-spinal, system, there results a motion, a movement. When the response is effected through the involuntary, or sympathetic, nervous system, there results a feeling or emotion. The cerebro-spinal system of nerves is thus commonly associated with voluntary, purposive acts; with consciousness, will, the *joyful and expanding emotions*, and brings the individual into relationship with the outer world; while the sympathetic system has to deal with nutrition and the preservation of the body and is associated with unconscious acts which, when they become conscious, we recognise as contracting *painful emotions*, such as fear or anger.

Important discoveries, made within recent years, prove that the sympathetic nervous system stimulates the secretion of the ductless or endocrine glands; and that their secretion, in turn, increases the sympathetic response and affects our emotions. These secretory glands are called ductless glands because there exists no visible duct (or tube) whereby their secretions may be conveyed away from the gland. The secretions formed are absorbed, indirectly, into the blood, through the cells of the gland and the walls of the lymph and blood vessels; and, after being discharged into the blood stream, they get carried to all the organs of the body, many of which they take effect upon—the effect varying with the particular organ and secretion.

Excess of certain glandular secretions can increase specific emotions, such as fear and anger—but they do not create them. The dispositions to them must be pre-existent. We all differ in our primary emotions, quite independently of the state of our internal organs and glandular secretions. These chemical and glandular theories have thrown some light on special mental disorders which are caused by such agencies, but they have not touched the great problems concerning mind and brain. However, as usual, enthusiasm following a new investigation often outstrips the limits of reasonableness and leads to such optimistic descriptions as LOUIS BERMAN has given in his book: *The Glands Regulating Personality* (1921).

THE ASCENT FROM THE UNCONSCIOUS TO SELF-CONSCIOUSNESS

Our inherited dispositions—our primary innate capacities, rudimentary emotions, and instinctive tendencies—are all *unconscious.* Only after their manifestation, by reflection on our impulses and conduct, do we become aware of them.

Besides the inherited tendencies, we all accumulate a vast number of experiences and acquisitions from our educators and the influence of our surroundings; and, since we can only be conscious of one thing at a time, all these impressions, of which we are made conscious by external sensations, as well as by the association of ideas, must be relegated to—what is called for convenience' sake—the *subconscious* mind.

We all see the same world objectively, but according to our subconscious and unconscious minds we look through different spectacles, and the scenery suggests to us different ideas. The inherited unconscious and the acquired subconscious elements form the basis of our character, and condition conduct to a far greater extent than the view of life that we express, and by which we believe that we are actuated. It is only on reflection after the act that most men realise the motive which prompted them to certain conduct. Many men are misers, ambitious, suspicious, conceited, and so forth, without being conscious of the fact; but their fellow-men know it.

It is the education of the conscious self which tends to uniformity in all civilised people. The subconscious self, however, which is built up out of that countless multitude of impressions, and their recurrence coming from the surroundings, customs, languages, national types, physical effects of climate, and many other sources, is widely different. They create a subconscious self in every person, and make him not merely a representative of his times, but produce in him the qualities peculiar to his country, to his race, and to the class in society to which he belongs, thus stamping him at once with their limitations and idiosyncrasies. For example, an educated Frenchman, German, and Englishman, may all have been brought up alike, so that ordinarily, in their views and manners, there is no distinction between them. But when, for any reason—emotional, for instance, or through depression or illness, or from a sudden surprise—their conscious self is weakened or fails them, their subconscious self asserts itself, and the national characteristics may appear, in spite of their uniform culture.

We have, then, two states of mind: the conscious or objective, and the subconscious or subjective. These distinctions, however, are made only for descriptive purposes. Indeed, there is no dividing line between them. As a rule, they work together; so that—whether we think, love, or are angry—we have always the feeling of *one personality*. Consciousness runs in personal streams, at all events so long as the brain is stable. As the brain grows, decays, or is influenced by various agents, so will consciousness vary; but the main character, the main self, always remains behind these variations.

Some psychologists argue that there is no subconsciousness; but we have no other expression for those experiences, thoughts, and emotions which are not in consciousness at any given moment. Whether we admit an absolute unconsciousness or a relative unconsciousness or subconsciousness, a subliminal consciousness, or a secondary consciousness, or a fringe of consciousness, does not matter much at the present stage, so long as we are agreed that past experiences are stored in another unknown region, or, at least, do not remain in consciousness, but are capable of being revived in consciousness.

Consciousness is only a phase of our psychical life, but not the psychical life itself. So far as there is consciousness, there is certainly mental activity; but it is not true that so far as there is mental activity, there is consciousness. There is a thousand times more below the surface of consciousness than there is above. We flatter ourselves that it is we who are thinking; whereas subconscious thinking goes on all the time. Mind and consciousness are therefore not synonymous or coextensive. During a particular conscious state all the rest of the mind is dormant. Consciousness knows only the result of the work done in the unknown laboratory beneath it.

Consciousness increases with the complexity of the nervous system. It develops gradually from subconsciousness to consciousness, and from consciousness to self-consciousness, that state in which we are able to control our thoughts in the very process of thinking.

Psychologists took some time in discovering that there is a relation between psychical activity and the brain; for consciousness does not reveal to us the existence of a brain, gives no information regarding the operations of the brain, or of the functions of any other internal organ. Man, in general, in the state of health, has no consciousness of the existence or uses of the brain; and in consequence of this want of consciousness, psychologists have for so long ascribed the phenomena of sensation, emotion, and thought exclusively to a spiritual entity which they have named—the mind.

But, as I have pointed out at the beginning of this chapter, we are not conscious even of having a mind; we are conscious only of mental states and acts.

The Development of the Human Mind

Man has made a slow, gradual ascent from a purely animal stage, but he is still largely under the control of the powerful instincts and appetites inherited from his prehistoric origin, and shares many qualities possessed by the lower animals.

No matter how low the animal in organisation, it is invariably imbued with the desire to live. We call it the *instinct of self-preservation.* Even the jelly-fish will protect itself when it thinks it is in danger of physical injury or destruction. If it were not for the instinct for self-preservation, we should never move out of the way of danger, never raise a hand to avert a fall or blow.

The animal and man alike cannot maintain life by merely protecting themselves against mechanical injury, but require food in order to exist. Hunger and thirst are the two painful sensations provided by nature to prompt the animal to go in search of food. We call this the *alimentary instinct.* The gratification of the eating and drinking impulse is a source of pleasure to the animal. The animal eats in order to maintain its existence, but it is not conscious of the reason.

In order to obtain food, carnivorous animals, and flesh-eating man, must kill other animals. Civilised man relegates this duty to a special section of the community; but he still hunts and kills for sport. From the biological standpoint the *combative instinct* is to be regarded as a normal mental attribute for the maintenance of existence, and many animals are provided with special weapons of offence and defence, in the shape of horns, claws, and the like.

The emotion attaching to the combative instinct is *anger*. It is an emotion necessary for protection from oppression and for self-defence. In order to defend, we must be strong enough to assail. The emotion of anger is aroused by anything that hampers or inhibits the activities of the individual. Unless controlled, it causes the combatant to assume a ferocious aspect, while at the same time it has the effect of liberating a flood of muscular energy needful for the ferocity of onslaught. Hunger causes the animal to become savage, and this, in a measure, is also true of man. All living nature is in deadly conflict. We must think, not of civilised man, but of man in the savage stage, when he had to fight for his bare existence.

Civilised man no longer depends so much on muscular strength, since money is to him the great protector of life, and, with it, he can even induce other men to do the fighting for him. Moreover, as soon as man lived in communities, he tried to diminish strife by instituting laws for the equal protection of all; but nations still fight for their existence, not merely for food for their people, but for such commodities as oil and coal.

Not all animals, however, are provided with the instruments for a fight. Consequently, nature has given them other means for self-defence, such as increased powers of locomotion in order to run or fly away. This must be done in time, and is accomplished by the emotion of *fear*. Such animals are timid, easily afraid; and this makes them alert to the slightest unusual happening, and equally quick to escape. It is fear, also, that urges the organism to avoid a previous danger, and therefore fear has a definite biological value. The intellectual application of fear produces caution. Without sufficient caution we should not see danger until it was too late. It would be difficult to be circumspect.

Animals frequently use strategy in attack, and concealment in defence. They may hide, or sham death. This cunning disposition is protective, because it suggests to the enemy that there is no adversary or prey, and it serves in place of courage. It makes the animal alert by a *feeling of suspicion* and distrustfulness; and, by arousing curiosity, stimulates it to examine objects to discover whether they are dangerous. Some animals are more cunning than others, and the same secretiveness is common to man, in whom it varies also in a marked degree. The reverse of suspicion is over-trustfulness.

As animals are not always able to secure food—food being scarce at certain periods of the year—certain species find it advantageous to collect and hoard it. Men hoard too, not only food, but money and other valuables, with which they can buy their necessities and luxuries. The *disposition to acquire* and hoard varies in degree congenitally.

Besides the instinct of self-preservation, nature is interested in the preservation of the species. Consequently, it has endowed all living beings with the tendency to propagate. The *sex instinct* is the most powerful of all the instincts.

Two beings unite in love; they live together; they found a home, just as the birds build a nest; and, in due course, there will be young ones. Then another disposition comes into force, one of affection for the helpless young —*parental love*—and the infant's affection for the parents—*filial love*.

A further disposition aroused is the attachment to the family settlement: the *love of home*. Where there are several children, and from the environment of other homes, there springs social life and *social attachment.*

Social life created the feelings connected with the personality. In a community some are born to lead—the self-confident and self-reliant. Others are content to follow and obey. The more energetic are created leaders and demand obedience from the rest. *Self-esteem,* in excess, may lead to pride, conceit, and arrogance. This feeling, when defective, causes under-estimation of self and of one's powers; and a lack of confidence, hindering the proper use of one's talents. Reliance on one's self gives resolute character, tenacity, firmness, strength of will.

Social life, moreover, necessitates adaptation to one's fellow-men and surroundings. It gives rise to the desire to please and excel, and thus ensures good conduct. It creates the *desire to gain approbation* and to avoid disapprobation, and thus lays the foundation of civility in intercourse.

Social life has developed also one great gift—that of *speech.* Speech, in its origin, is an expression of feeling. The first utterances of infancy are simple ejaculations of like or dislike. Words are formed when these ejaculations are uttered in particular sounds for particular objects.

Now let us pass to the intellectual dispositions proper. First of all, curiosity is aroused by what is unfamiliar, and prompts to investigation, and investigation leads to knowledge. To satisfy our curiosity and to gain knowledge, we must possess the power of observation and perception. Seeing is not perceiving. In order to perceive we must *actively* look, not only *passively* see. The perceptions are stored in memory, and may be recalled. Without proper perception there can be no memory.

Both *perception* and *memory* are highly complex qualities.

Some people have an excellent memory for words, but not for figures. Others possess a good memory for facts and events, but not for dates and the lapse of time. Again, some can remember the forms of objects seen better than others; but not their dimensions, colour, or the place of their situation.

In addition to observation and memory, we have the power of *reasoning* upon the knowledge gained, by a process of induction and a process of deduction; and these processes vary in degree in different men. Some draw conclusions by a simple act of comparison; others base their judgment on what has gone before. Again, some people are better at observation than reasoning, whilst others are the reverse. Reasoning needs the combining of recollections and gives an inquiring mind, one that is not satisfied with the mere fact that things exist, but seeks the reason why.

The capacities we have described so far are capacities for intellectual *processes*, rather than abilities. Every man possesses, in addition, special aptitudes, native gifts for certain lines of activity; as, for example, mathematics, music, mechanics, and the like, in varying degree.

There are still two mental powers to be mentioned, as to which opinion varies whether they are intellectual or instinctive. The one is constructive ability; the other imitation.

Constructive ability is certainly innate and exists in animals. But the animal never improves upon its constructions, whereas man is constantly progressing in his designs. The element underlying construction in man is, doubtless, manual dexterity; but in its more developed stage it is entirely mental.

The other mental quality, the power of *imitation*, may be confined to imitation of work, or to the manners and tastes of others; or may be facial dexterity, as in mimicry. Children imitate their elders, and thus is preserved the continuity of manners and tastes from one generation to another.

Next, there is developed the power of *imagination*—largely by the power of speech, which enables us to think in the abstract.

The thirst for knowledge of the educated thinker is not contented with the defective acquaintance with the outer world: an acquaintance obtained through our imperfect sense organs. He endeavours to build up the sense impressions into valuable knowledge. He transforms them into perceptions and apperceptions, and combines them into presentations, by association. Finally, by a further concentration of the groups of presentations, he attains to connected knowledge. But this knowledge remains defective and unsatisfactory until the imagination supplements the inadequate power of combination of the intelligence, and, by the association of stored-up images, unites the isolated elements into a connected whole. Although imagination enters into every field of human experience, and busies itself with every line of human interest, yet all its activities can be classed under two different types. They are (1) reproductive, and (2) creative imagination.

Imagination enables us to endow certain objects with greater excellence than others, and this has given rise to the sense of beauty, *the aesthetic sense*, so essential to poets and artists. Imagery is man's creative faculty. We create, in thought-form, whatever we have the power to imagine. By the faculty of imagery we build up, in our minds, forms of beauty, of poetry, fiction, drama, music; indeed, of all that is sublime and lovable and worth realising.

By the power of his imagination man placed himself in the position of others, and felt with them—sympathised with their joys and sorrows Such sympathy gave rise to the feelings of charity and generosity, and the *ethical sentiments*. Ideals of social life were thus created which resulted in mutual assistance—altruism—becoming a principle of social conduct.

Everyone acts according to his own disposition, but those deeds are most praiseworthy which are for the good of the greatest number. Thus, advancing intelligence and social life established a moral code for all individuals within the same group. Moral conduct is conduct that serves the common interest. We estimate those things as right that are generally approved; and many people never go beyond this stage. They accept the conventional morality that they find prevalent. Their judgment of what is right is based on the approval of others.

Moral codes have varied at different times and in different parts of the earth; but they all have one principle in common: "Do not do to others what you would not wish they should do to you." Moral conduct has to be trained; whereas the animal instincts manifest themselves spontaneously In the lowest stage, the greatest force to good conduct is the fear of consequences, i.e. fear of punishment. It requires considerable development before we get the sentiment of right and wrong, the sentiment of duty and conscience.

The power of imagination has also led to the evolution of the sentiments of wonder, awe, faith, and veneration—the so called *religious sentiments*. Reverence for exalted powers, faith and belief in them, and the unexplained phenomena of life and creation, led men to the recognition of a Universal Creator, to the worship of an Almighty, and the different religions of mankind.

We have seen, then, that man possesses a variety of mental powers, which have different functions to perform, different duties to discharge, and between which there obtain certain relations and connections—some ranking higher, some lower

—yet all useful and necessary in their proper place. These primary mental powers exist in all men; their difference is one of degree only; for example, one man has more apprehension and less aggressiveness; another, more self-reliance and less veneration; a third, more affection and less greed, than some other person. We start life unequally, because of the difference in our surrounding circumstances. Education, law, public opinion, tend to repress impulses and to produce uniform conduct; but nature will out. That our dispositions are innate, and not the result of education and training—though these can and do produce certain habits and complexes—is evident from the contrasts we observe between members of the same family. Let wealth and power be distributed as may be, nevertheless the more industrious, the more artful, and the more gifted of men will have the best chance to rise to superiority. Only the animal is contented: at least so long as it gets its food. Man is rarely ever contented; he desires possessions, power, influence. *Our innate dispositions give us realisable potentiality, and environment makes the realisation of potentiality possible.* There are many geniuses in the world who remain undeveloped and obscure for lack of opportunity; and there are also many imbeciles whose defects are hidden because they are never called upon to do anything requiring intelligence.

The Development of the Human Brain

We have just analysed the human mind and mentioned a variety of instinctive dispositions, emotional tendencies, and intellectual abilities; but *not all of them, or perhaps not any of them, are really elementary.* From the physiological standpoint, they are very complex. They are certainly capable of combining into still more complex mental states and capacities; and *though we may find an area in the brain to which they are related, it is only the elements which are located there.* Just as natural substances become by synthesis transformed into other substances, so the mental elements, which depend on the functional activity of groups of brain cells, are actually transformed by combination into mental complexes different from those elements from which they started. The synthetic product of our thoughts is not the same as the elements; as little as water is identical with two elements of hydrogen and one element of oxygen. It is neither the one nor the other, but a new product.

Various physiologists, regarding mind as an entity, have endeavoured to solve the problem of its relation to the brain. In the opinion of some, thoughts were merely secretions of the brain; though no secreting organ ever creates that which it secretes. There is nothing in the constitution of the brain cell that can be converted into ideas. No mechanical or chemical theory can explain the creation of an original thought—say, the creation of a poem, or a beautiful piece of music, before it is written down. If man were purely a piece of mechanism, he could not be at the same time a spectator. Therefore, the modern view, which regards psychical activities as functions of the brain, is more moderate. But this view, too, does not explain how it is that we are able consciously to control mental manifestations, and even to manifest tendencies opposed to our natural inclinations. Consequently, a number of physiologists content themselves with assuming that psychical activities run parallel with brain activities, without attempting to solve how they act upon each other.

All these views fail to explain what starts the impulse in

the brain cell. Assuming it is a chemical process, what made it occur just then and in that particular way? What is the peculiarity of the brain cell that transforms a sensation into an idea? What enables it to receive the sound of words and respond with feelings of love or anger? How can the light-waves which strike the retina on the reading of—say, the written words of a telegram—account for the exhibition of emotional forces, different persons being differently affected by the same cause?

Chemico-physical changes in the nerve cells are supposed by some to be the *cause* of consciousness, and of everything which goes to make up the human mind. Thus that eminent American scientist, JACQUES LOEB (*The Mechanistic Conception of Life*, Chicago, 1912), believed that life's wishes and hopes, efforts and struggles, disappointments and sufferings are amenable to a physico-chemical analysis, because he could explain animal tropism, i.e. the tendency of certain animals to fly or creep to the light, on such a basis, He considered this tendency to be instinctive, and, being able to explain the one instinct, he could see no reason why the whole of man's inner life should not receive a physico-chemical explanation. But, in my opinion, the tendency of certain animals to go instinctively to a source of light is not a universal or a primitive instinct.

Loeb has undoubtedly made some valuable contributions to our knowledge of the behaviour of animals, and made an original study of the conduct of winged plant-lice—but surely it is a long way from plant-lice to the complex behaviour of man! For all we know, the plant-louse may have some noble inspirations, and as regards food, reproduction, etc., may have instincts identical with man; still, man is so far removed from the insect, that no correct deductions can be drawn from one to the other.

That, however, was not the opinion of Loeb and the school he represented. On the contrary, all that is noble in man was considered by Loeb purely mechanical. "Our instincts", he said, "are hereditary, as is the form of the body, and we obey them 'machine-like'—for we are *compelled* to do so. . . . We struggle for justice and truth since we are instinctively compelled to see our fellow-beings happy." How many men did Loeb believe to be struggling for justice and truth? And what is the physico-chemical explanation of this struggle? "Not only", said he, "is the mechanistic conception of life compatible with ethics: it seems the only conception of life which can lead to an understanding of the source of ethics." May I ask what ethics can there be in compulsion? On a physico-chemical basis practically all men should be virtuous, for they are so organised, and their actions could be foretold.

Our concern in this book is not with "mind", but with the various mental activities, and we shall try to trace their localisation in the brain. This has been attempted on a large scale for the past sixty years; yet it will be shown that, whilst immense progress has been made in nearly every other branch of medical research, we are, as yet, no nearer to the solution of this problem, which is one of the greatest interest and the most far-reaching importance.

We shall deal in the next chapter with the electrical excitation and experimental destruction of the brains of animals; and the reasons why these investigations have failed. In Chapter III we shall survey the discoveries made in the microscopical anatomy of the brain and the conflicting theories to which they have given rise. But this much we may say here, that, whatever method is adopted for the discovery of the mental functions of the brain, we shall fail, so long as we remain under the influence of antiquated notions of the mind derived from self-introspection. What is needed is a biological and comparative study of the mind, and tracing the concurrent development of the brain from the lowest animal to the mighty genius of man.

For the benefit of those not acquainted with brain anatomy,

I may as well explain, at the outset, that the human brain consists of two equal hemispheres, each of which has an outer portion—the cortex—grey in colour, and arranged in folds (convolutions), and consisting of several layers of microscopic cells, varying in design according to locality, and an inner white portion, consisting of nerve fibres, connecting the different parts of the surface, and communicating with the central basal structures and also with the spinal cord.

Now, it is a universally accepted fact that this grey matter (the cortex or outer rind of the brain, which is in contact with the inner surface of the skull) is the structure through the medium of which all mental operations take place.

We think and feel, rejoice and weep, love and hate, hope and fear, plan and destroy, trust and suspect, all through the agency of the brain cortex. Its cells record all the events, of whatever nature, which transpire within the individual's sphere of existence, not merely as concerns the intellectual knowledge acquired, but, likewise, the emotions passed through, and the passions indulged in. *We can only manifest our intellectual aptitudes, moral dispositions, and tendencies to self-preservation, through the mechanism of brain with which we happen to be endowed, and according to the sort of experience we have accumulated.* Hence, though the primitive mental powers and fundamental anatomical parts of the brain of all men are the same, we all vary according to the mental predispositions and brain-types we have inherited, and the early education that we received.

True, in some of the lower animals the psychic life is not inseparably bound to the cerebral hemispheres; still, in the case of the higher mammals, and especially in the case of man, the connection undoubtedly exists.

In the lowest vertebrates, the fishes, we get for the first time a rudimentary cerebrum and cerebellum; but as yet no cortex of the brain, except over the olfactory lobes, that

PLATE II

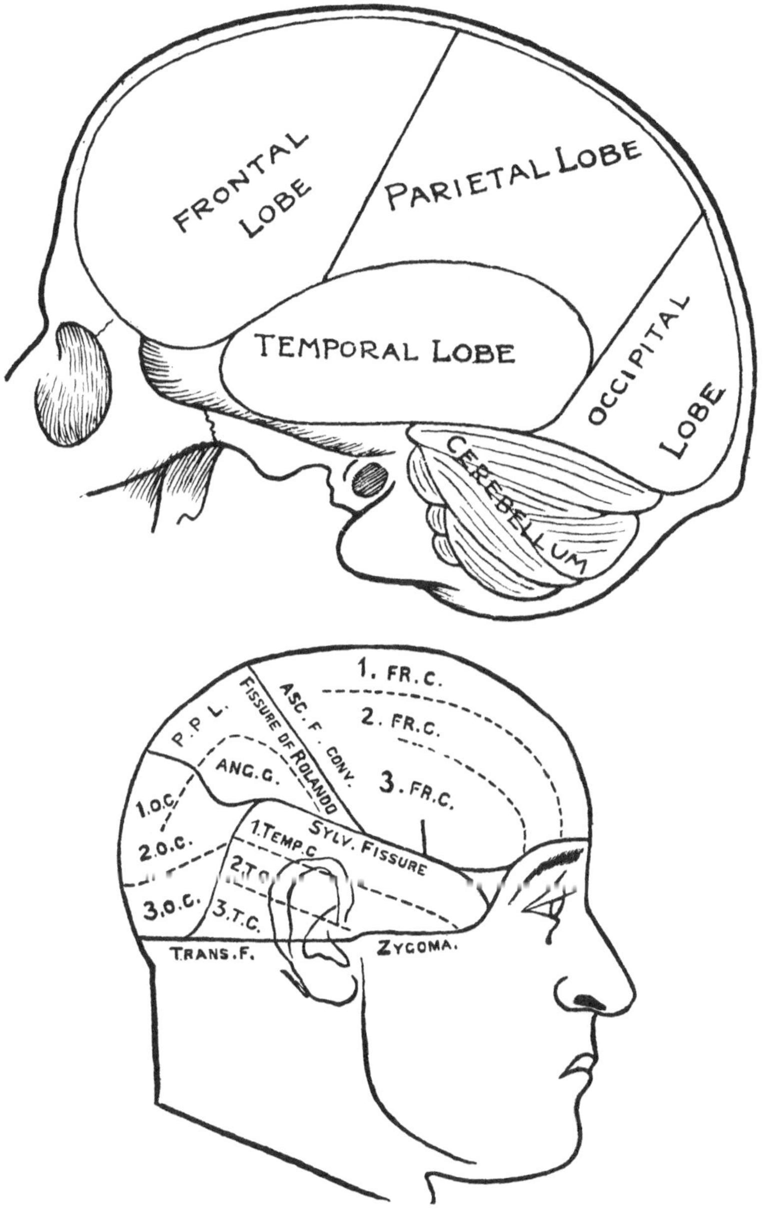

TWO DIAGRAMS OF CRANIO-CEREBRAL RELATIONS

part of the brain related to smell. In the amphibia we get a larger cortex, a membranous roof extending over the basal ganglia, but still the olfactory cortex is the most prominent; and in the reptiles, we get a still larger one. In the case of mammals, the highest class of vertebrates, we find proper cerebral hemispheres and an ever-increasing cortex, with its highest development in man.

Not only does the whole brain increase in size, but in the higher mammals the cortex grows so rapidly—as compared with the deeper parts—that it becomes crumpled, that is to say, convoluted. These convolutions greatly augment the surface of the cortex for the increase of the number of brain cells. Man has three times as many cortical neurons as any other animal. Whilst a rabbit's brain has still a very smooth surface, the brain of carnivorous, pachydermatous, and ruminant animals is convoluted; yet the convolutions are not yet arranged in definite lobes, as in the human brain, but lie in successive tiers around the Sylvian fissure.

Since the brain becomes more convoluted, and the convolutions more distinct and numerous, as we ascend the scale o fthe animal kingdom, we must assume that the essential differences obtaining in the brain structure correspond to decided differences in its functions and have some relation to the variety of animal instincts. If it be admitted that these instincts are hereditary, then it may as well be admitted that they are due to some peculiarity in the brain structure.

Moreover, it will be shown in this book that *the parts of the brain which we have in common with the lower animals have corresponding mental functions; and those parts which are distinctly human, serve for the manifestations of the higher intellectual processes and abilities and man's most exalted sentiments.*

Just as in animals that possess an extraordinary sense of smell there is a relatively enormous development of the olfactory bulbs, so in men, whose chief characteristic is an extraordinary degree of some special mental power, only that part of the brain which is concerned with its manifestation will be found remarkably developed, as compared with the remainder of the cortex of the brain.

Admitting a multiplicity of centres in the brain, we can at once understand how it is that one man may excel and be excellent in one thing and stupid in another; just the same as a man may have strong eyesight and be very deaf; or a fine sense of scent and no power of hearing. A little observation shows us that some people, apart from all training, have a decided capacity for certain pursuits. Some excel in history, others in geography; whilst some are undoubtedly born mathematicians, musicians, painters, or poets. If the same portion of brain matter were engaged in all studies equally, then a man who excels in mathematics should be equally able to excel in drawing or music; but we find great metaphysicians who cannot learn the multiplication table; colourists who cannot draw; and other examples of one-sided talent. Most of us are wholly devoid in some mental power, and no training will enable us to acquire skill in it.

If intellectual qualities are inborn and require specific brain structures, we may conclude the same of the instincts and emotions. Do we not find that children show different dispositions to fear, anger, love, etc., in different degrees, quite independent of intellectual influence; and do we not find, sometimes, that the best of training fails to curb the natural inclinations? If we do not admit that these inclinations are due to peculiarities of brain-organisation, how can we explain them? We should have to assume that all character is due to education and experience, in which case no reliance could be placed on the actions of men.

Infant prodigies are usually quite as childish as other children in everything but the talent by which they are particularly distinguished. On the other hand, in idiocy and imbecility, the individual is exceedingly deficient in most of the intellectual powers, and frequently in some of the moral sentiments; but yet may possess a few of them in considerable vigour. It is not uncommon to find in feeble-minded children one remarkable faculty—for music, imitation, drawing, memory for numbers, dates, events, etc.—without comprehending a single abstract idea; or they may show some special instinct, and yet manifest no other power to any appreciable extent; which would be impossible were there no distinct centres in the brain.

Further, the existence of such evidence as will be given in this book, as, for instance, that of injuries of the head affecting, not infrequently, one or more of the mental powers, while others remain perfectly sound—renders the supposition far from unreasonable that the different portions of the cerebral hemispheres have different functions allotted to them. Similarly, circumscribed lesions due to the growth of tumours, the effects of haemorrhage, etc., often give rise to definite mental changes; and, whenever the injury, or the compression, affects the same locality, the same mental symptoms can be observed.

Last, but not least, we have the observations of numerous investigators, showing that certain regions of the cerebrum are distinguished from other regions by broad difference in structure. Not only does the structure in different convolutions assume, to a greater or lesser extent, a variety or modifications, but even different parts of the same convolution may vary, with regard either to the arrangement or the relative size of their cells. These structural differences must be correlated with some difference of function. The group of cells the function of which is purely intellectual, cannot possibly have the same construction as a group of cells which serves for emotional manifestation. The two may be united by association fibres, so that one may rouse the other; but the function of each group of cells must be distinct.

Brain investigations have hitherto been carried out on the wrong assumption that mind and intellect are equivalent, and that the brain is, therefore, primarily an intellectual organ; whereas the truth is that *the brain is, primarily, an organ for the adaptation of the individual to his surroundings, in order to preserve his existence*; and it is from this point of view that new investigations should be commenced.

It will also be shown that many investigators have returned to the view that the brain acts, more or less, as a uniform organ; and even those who admit the possibility of multiple centres in the brain do so only with reference to movement and sensation (motor and sensory centres), but deny mental localisation.

The cerebral origin of the instincts has, so far, been totally neglected; and the emotions which arise from them have also received little attention by physiologists. The question must now be seriously asked: "Are the primary emotions and instinctive tendencies, which we have in common with animals, connected with the cortex (the outer rind of the brain), certain basal ganglia, or have they no connection with the brain at all?" This is a vital question, the solution of which is absolutely essential for real progress in psychology and cerebral physiology and for the proper understanding and treatment of mental disorders.

Is the whole brain the organ of the intellect, or is it restricted to either the frontal, parietal, occipital, or temporal lobes? We shall quote opinions of eminent authorities in support of each one of these areas.

There is also considerable confusion as to the meaning of the term "intellect". When, for example, RONCORONI says, "We cannot admit that the more highly evolved faculties have any limited seat, nor can we accept as admissible those theories which localise intelligence, memory, will, or consciousness in the frontal lobes", he is quite right. The "faculties" mentioned cannot be localised. Intelligence is not identical with intellect. It is the property of the entire brain. An individual's intelligence is the ability to learn, to profit by experience, to react efficiently; in other words, his competence and facility in dealing in a practical manner with his environment, or, in a wider meaning—his capacity of common sense. Nor would anyone think of locating will, or consciousness; and, as regards memory, every part of the brain is endowed with it. Memory varies according to its application. There is the memory for words, numbers, tunes, faces, for facts and events, etc. Every fundamental propensity also has its own memory. For example, some men have a good memory for money transactions, others for injuries received, others for impressions of dangers; and so forth, according to their instinctive and emotional dispositions.

Neurologists do not usually observe mental changes; at least not systematically, by means of a proper psychological plan. That is why they tell us that the brain acts as a uniform organ. But alienists, as specialists in mental disease, should not be guided by them. If the insanities are essentially disorders of the brain, as all must admit in a final analysis of the subject, and if the brain is recognised, not as an organ, all parts of which are necessary to every function—or an organ, one part of which is sufficient for all functions—but as an assemblage or confederation of separate organs or centres, each of which is independent, or at least autonomous —it follows that the facts and principles of cerebral localisation must play an important rôle in the solution of psychiatric problems, and, especially, in the elucidation of mental symptoms, and the causation, duration, and prognosis of the different types of insanity.

CHAPTER II

THE RESULTS OF EXPERIMENTAL PHYSIOLOGY

One of the reasons for the lack of knowledge of the mental functions of the brain is that too much reliance has been placed on the experiments performed in laboratories on the brains of living animals. For fifty years (1821–71) medical opinion and the opinion of philosophers and psychologists was dominated by the results of FLOURENS's experiments, which seemed to prove that the brain is a uniform organ as regards its functions. Flourens held that the whole of the cerebral mass is homogeneous, that nothing prevents the functions of one part being transferred to another, and that so long as one little part is left, the intellectual faculties and consciousness will still remain. (*Experimental Researches into the Properties and Functions of the Nervous System in Vertebrate Animals*, Paris, 1822—a report which had obtained the prize of the French Academy.)

Flourens took a live pigeon for his investigation, and removed the brain in successive stages. After cutting the "soul" from his fowl bit by bit (the expression used by his contemporaries), he found that the mental faculties and consciousness were preserved, and from his observation of a pigeon's brain he drew the deduction that man's cerebral mass, too, was homogeneous in function. Later, he used other low-grade animals, and applied small metal balls to the surface of the brain, letting them slowly sink through. The balls, in every case, forced their way, in course of time, right through to the base of the brain, without resulting in any disturbance of function whatever. After these ingenious experiments, there was no longer any question that the brain acted as a single organ, and contained no centres of special function.

Flourens started his investigation with a preconceived notion of the unity of mind, and found what he expected to find, namely, that the brain, too, was a unity. As in the case of other physiologists, the results, only too often, are according to the psychological views of the observer. Flourens's indivisibility of the "ego" appealed to the philosophers of his time. The idea that the brain might be parcelled out into distinct areas of differentiated activities was thenceforth habitually stigmatised as contemptibly ridiculous, and unworthy of scientific consideration. Flourens's opinion dominated the medical world for fifty years, to the exclusion of all progress in our knowledge of brain functions.

There were experts, in those days, who brought forward evidence supporting the theory of the localisation of mental functions in the brain; but they only met with boycott or abuse in face of such "scientific" proof to the contrary; and that by men who perhaps had never seen a brain dissected, for the real experts are few in number.

When, in 1871, these experiments were proved by Hitzig and Fritsch to be conducted on animals too low in the scale of cerebral organisation, and localisation was admitted, it was still not recognised that we cannot draw conclusions from the behaviour of a dumb animal—anaesthetised in many cases—as to the complicated mental organisation of man. Electrical stimulation, under the conditions in which such animals are placed, will give rise to sensations, to which they will respond with movements. All we can expect, therefore, is to discover sensory and motor centres. At first, nearly the whole brain was mapped out with these centres (Ferrier, 1873); then it was discovered that the motor field was restricted to the two central convolutions of the brain (Horsley and Beevor, 1885); later, only the anterior central

Plate III

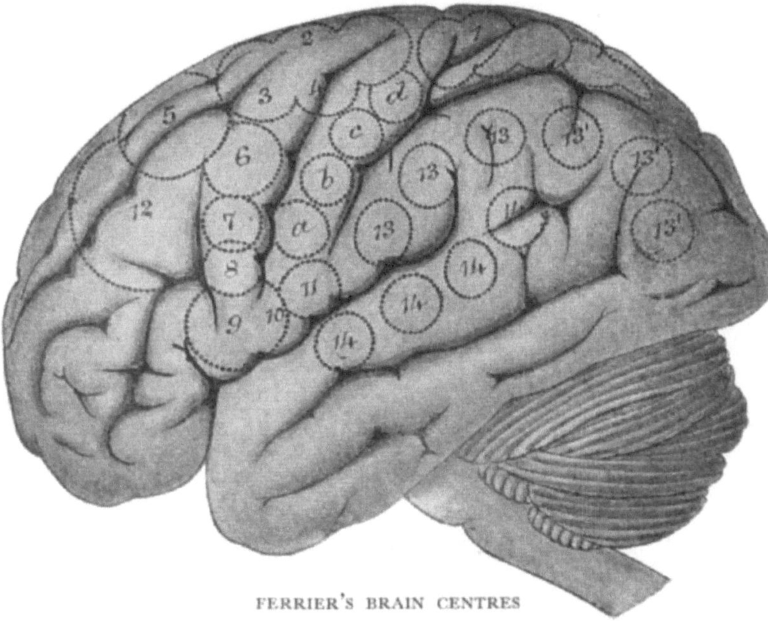

FERRIER'S BRAIN CENTRES

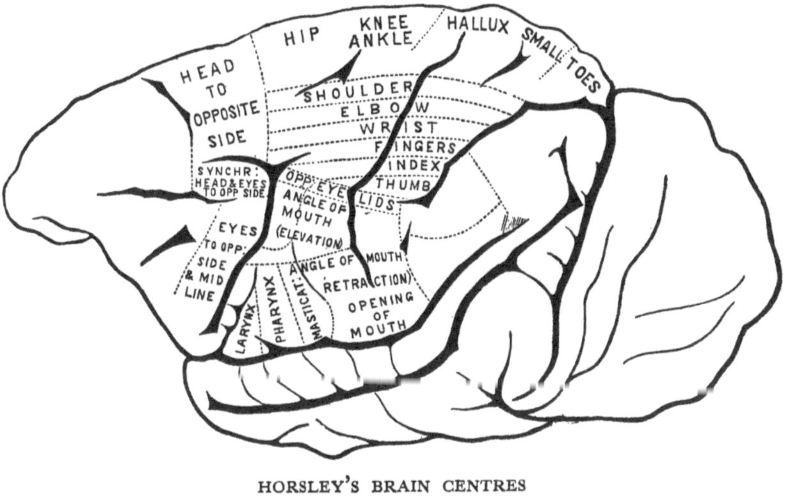

HORSLEY'S BRAIN CENTRES

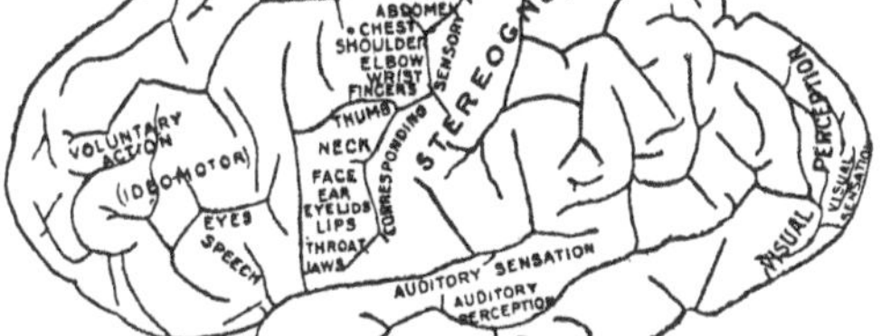

SHERRINGTON'S BRAIN CENTRES

convolution was declared to respond with movements (SHERRINGTON and GRÜNBAUM, 1901). Later still, it was admitted that these centres might, after all, not be cortical, but sub-cortical; for the "movements return after complete destruction of the motor area" (SIR VICTOR HORSLEY, *British Medical Journal*, 1909). CHARLTON BASTIAN wrote a reply in the same journal, agreeing that "the true motor centres are lower down in the brain and spinal cord".

Now, it is interesting to observe the psychological effect of a doctrine that happens to be fashionable at the moment. It fills the mind with preconceptions, so that investigators are apt to see what they expect to see.

Although the posterior central convolution was proved by SHERRINGTON to have nothing to do with the motor area, yet BASTIAN and HORSLEY (*Brain*, Vol. III) had previously declared that they had seen it atrophied in cases of "congenital absence of one hand"; so had WIGLESWORTH (*Journal of Mental Science*, 1886) in the case of an "Old Amputation of the left Upper Arm"; and CAMPBELL (*Histological Studies on the Localisation of Cerebral Functions*, Cambridge, 1905) also claimed to have observed histological changes in the posterior central convolution, in three cases of amputation of a leg, and in three cases of amputation of an arm. Other cases are: GOWERS (*Brain*, 1878) in congenital defect of left arm; CHUQUET (*Bull. de la Soc. Anat.*, 1876) in amputation of left arm six years before death; and BOYER, who saw both anterior and posterior central convolutions on the left side atrophied, in amputation of left arm thirty-one years before death. Then we have LANDOUZY (*Bull. de la Soc. Anat.*, 1877), who found the left post-central convolution atrophied in injury to right leg, which rendered it useless; and OUDIN (*Revue Mens.*, 1878), who found the left anterior and posterior central convolutions atrophied on both sides, in infantile paralysis (!) of right leg. On the other hand, CHARCOT (*Soc. de Biol.*, 1878) denied the possibility of these observations.

ROLANDO should be remembered here, as having been the first to excite the surface of the brains of animals electrically, as long ago as 1828. He believed that the white substance. not the grey, produced particular movements, but he did not define them. FLOURENS, too, did not think the cortex to be thus excitable, and held that the current travelled down to the structures at the base of the brain, and thence to the spinal cord.

The ascending frontal convolution (pre-central convolution) was mapped out (by the experimenters mentioned) in cortical points, set in ladder-like fashion. At the extreme upper end are the centres for the leg; those for the toes and ankle being actually on the mesial aspect of the hemispheres. The knee and hip are followed by the trunk; and below this comes the shoulder, elbow, wrist, fingers, and thumb, in this order. The eyelids, mouth, tongue, and larynx follow; whilst, just in front of the hand area, is a special centre devoted to the conjugate movements of the eyes and head in rotating to the opposite side.

Yet it is now admitted that when the ascending frontal convolution is removed entirely, there follows only a temporary paralysis of the opposite side, with perfect recovery.

SHERRINGTON removed the whole of the face region of the cortex in a young chimpanzee, without even a transitory paralysis of either face, jaw, tongue, or larynx, which are supposed to have their centres in this area; on the contrary, the chimpanzee became more grimacing and noisy than before.

LASHLEY removed by ablation the entire cerebral cortex of rats, and found no signs of localisation of motor functions.

As early as 1891, E. H. BENNETT, of the University of Dublin, exhibited the brain of a patient whose death had been caused by the growth of a large tumour, which involved a very considerable area of the cerebral cortex, "but never during life was there any paralysis of the limbs".

BASTIAN described the motor area as the "kinaesthetic" area

(*Brain*, 1887) and as "a purely sensory area" (*British Medical Journal*, 1909); in other words, as an area for the sensory appreciation of muscular movements.

The post-central convolution was supposed to contain the centres for the more discriminating functions of sensibility. GRAHAM BROWN destroyed it in a chimpanzee without the animal manifesting any signs of disability, not seeming to have lost any sensory function. He then removed the left motor area as well; but after a fortnight's paralysis, the monkey recovered all his movements. Consequently, he came to the conclusion that "the experimental evidence gives no grounds for the supposition of the localisation of function of voluntary movement in the 'motor' area, as distinguished from any other part of the cortex".

MARION HINES wrote more recently: "The diagrams of local representation of function in the cerebral cortex, so prevalent in the last part of the nineteenth century, have gradually become dimmer, until, finally, point localisation has disappeared, even from the motor cortex, under the careful experimental analysis of Leyton, Sherrington, and Graham Brown. Only the projection of the retina upon the calcarine region now remains."

Yet even this last statement by Hines (with reference to the localisation of the sense of sight) is now denied by some. For instance, LOEB (*Pflüger's Archiv.*, Vol XXXIV), who had experimentally destroyed the entire visual sphere, found that no marked disturbances of sight were produced, even by the most extensive lesion of the occipital lobes; and LUCIANI and TAMBURINI agreed with him.

GUDDEN (*Neurologisches Centralblatt*, 1885) extirpated the whole occipital lobe in young rabbits, and found that they could still see very well. He had also removed the motor spheres in cats; but after a few hours they showed no motor disturbance. He concluded with the remark that he had little faith in the charts in which different centres were put down, as on a map.

According to Dr. JAMES COLLIER (*British Medical Journal*, January 11, 1930), a very great part of the visual cortex may be destroyed in man with little lowering of the visual faculty. "Visual disorientation", he says, "has always, in my experience, resulted from a bilateral lesion of the *white matter*, severing the transcortical path running forward from the occipital lobes."

Dr. Collier does not believe, either, in that big area of the temporal lobes which we see mapped out in textbook-diagrams for *hearing*. He says (in the same report): "The faculty of hearing is only disturbed in mass by a lesion of a very small area of the cortex of the temporal region (Heschl's gyrus), and then only when the lesion is bilateral." An animal trained to react in a certain way to a given noise can still do so correctly after the extirpation of the auditory cortical areas, and can still be trained to take its food at an auditory signal.

SCHAFER (*Proceedings of the Royal Society*, 1887) had already disputed the existence of the centre for hearing in the temporal lobes, for the reason that all his and Professor Brown's experiments on a large number of monkeys left their hearing unimpaired.

Dr. Collier holds that sensory effects are produced only by lesions of the white matter of the hemispheres, causing severance of fibres which establish connections between different parts of the cortex. But, if neither motor nor sensory areas are cortical—as has been believed hitherto—this leaves the grey matter of the brain, i.e. the cortex, free for mental functions. That, however, is not the view of Dr. Collier, who, realising the failure of experimental physiology, now considers the cerebral cortex to act as a whole, thus reverting to Flourens's view. We are back again where we were a hundred years ago, and it would seem that the laborious and extensive experiments on animals have been in vain. Let me quote Dr. Collier's own words:

"The experimental physiologists of to-day have laid down that the motor cortex is only so called by them, because it is more excitable than the rest of the cortex, and that, even in this region, liability of function, facilitation, and deviation of response, are much more characteristic features than is localisation; and that there must be other mechanisms than this precentral cortex, which act directly upon the lower mechanism by means of direct descending fibres; and that normal motor activation takes place through descending fibres from many parts of the cortex; and that, *in complex motor activity the cerebral cortex acts as a whole,* though the activity of some parts of it may be accentuated and of other parts depressed; and that the activity of any one part of the cortex is conditioned by the balance of innumerable activities which proceed from other parts of the cortex. *The physiologists have abandoned the localisation of function within the cerebral cortex*; and this position is in accord with the clinical evidence in man. *It is obvious that each region of the cerebral cortex must be of equal functional importance* in the make-up of the perfect animal."

A similar opinion was expressed long ago by Goltz (*Archiv. für Psychiatrie,* Vol. XXIV), namely, that every section of the brain, independently of the others, is connected with all the voluntary muscles and with all the sensory nerves of the body. It took thirty years of experiments to justify Goltz's original criticism (*Verrichtungen des Grosshirns,*

1881), that "It is not possible, by extirpating any amount of the substance of the cortex, on either side, or on both sides, to produce a permanent laming of any muscle of the body, or a total loss of sensibility in any of its parts".

The *British Medical Journal*, in a leading article commenting upon Dr. Collier's observations (January 11, 1930), wrote: "It appears probable that anatomy is reaching the end of its great contributions to neurology, and that we are entering upon an era which will be characterised by the development of neuro-physiological and neuro-psychological concepts in which *localisation of function will play little or no part.*"

Another investigator, Dr. Bruggia (quoted in the same article) will also have nothing to do with the localisation of functions in the brain. He refers to this conception as "the seduction of all seductions", to which so many have gone under. He is said to have put forward, at the end of his book of nearly two hundred pages, adequate and convincing proofs that in the nervous system "there are no centres of local functions".

Ferrier, the British pioneer of experimental brain physiology (with whom, as his clinical assistant, I had many discussions), knew the limitations of experiments on animal brains carried out for the discovery of the complex mental functions of man. In his own words:

"There is, perhaps, no subject in physiology of greater importance, and more general interest, than the functions of the brain, and there are few which present to experimental investigation conditions of greater intricacy and complexity. No one who has attentively studied the results of the labours of the numerous investigators in this field of research can help being struck by the want of harmony, and even positive contradictions, among the conclusions which apparently the same experiments and the same facts have led to in different hands. And, when the seemingly well-established facts of experimentation on the brains of the lower animals are compared with those of clinical observations and morbid anatomy in man, the discord between them is frequently so great as to lead many to the opinion that physiological investigation on the lower animals is little calculated to throw light on the functions of the human brain."

Yet, notwithstanding his own caution, his researches, at the outset, were greeted with enthusiastic leading articles in the medical journals, prophesying wonderful developments for his discoveries. It was confidently anticipated that "they would solve man's moral and spiritual mysteries", and that "the nature and causes of insanity would speedily be laid bare". Needless to say, these hopes have not been realised. And, to this day, Ferrier's later warning has been completely ignored. I refer to his address to the Congress of American Physicians and Surgeons in 1888 (*Transactions*, Vol. I), when he said:

"Though our knowledge of the functions of the brain, and of the principles of diagnosis of cerebral disease, has made enormous strides of late years, and has rendered possible the brilliant surgical achievements of which we have heard this evening, *we must not imagine that we really know much about the brain after all.* Though we can point to the portion of the brain concerned with the movements of the foot, the head, the mouth, etc., to that portion of the brain with which we see, or hear, or feel, and determine with a fair degree of accuracy the seat and kind of disease which invades the cerebral cortex, yet there are portions of the cortex which are to us still practically a *terra incognita*—and even with respect to the regions which I have alluded to, there are still considerable differences of opinion, which, though not materially affecting the diagnosis of cerebral disease, are yet of no little importance in relation to a true conception of the mechanism of brain function. For, *behind sensory and motor centres, there lie also all those functions which constitute mental phenomena*, a true correlation of which, with their material substrata, is even of greater importance, both theoretically and practically, than the mere determination of their physiological significance and the effects of irritative or destructive lesions. The sympathies between the different parts of the nervous system are so numerous, and so intricate, that it is often impossible to determine between the effects which are the necessary consequences of a particular injury and those which result from sympathy. If we add to these the difficulties arising from the possibility of deciding how much of the effect is attributable to the shock given to the whole animal system by the very severe wounds of other parts, and how much is due to the mutilation of the brain itself, our hopes of success will be very moderate. And *while we know so little of the functions of the primitive mental faculties as still to be disputing their number and nature, it seems to us little short of absurd to expect to discover which of them has disappeared.*"

When I first witnessed Horsley's experiments, over forty years ago, I pointed out (Anthropological Institute, 1889, and British Association Meetings, 1889 and 1890) that the effect of an experimental lesion, whether by electrical stimulation, or by destruction of a certain area of the surface of the brain, cannot be restrained to that portion only, on which the experiment was performed, but invariably penetrates deeper layers, and gives rise to disturbances at a distance. This is now admitted. I also pointed out, at the time, that these experiments had resulted in the location of centres for sensation and movement, but that the mind, which makes use of those centres, had escaped notice. Experimenters had succeeded, for instance, in locating a brain area for the movement of the hand, but had ignored the mind, which directed these movements for a definite end. Furthermore, I said that man had, in proportion to his body, a much larger and infinitely more complicated brain than the lower animals; although he had nothing like the amount of muscular energy, and acuity of senses which many of them possess. Consequently, it was fantastic to expect a solution of the working of the human brain—even that of the ordinary man, not to speak of great philosophers, scientists, poets, and artists—from the stimulation or destruction of bits of the cerebral tissue of a monkey, dog, or cat.

In my opinion too much has been made of the results of experimental physiology. Without a knowledge of the elements of the mind, and of the reciprocal influence of the various anatomically differentiated parts of the brain, all experiments on the cerebrum of animals, for the discovery of its functions, may be compared to the gropings of a blind man. *Experiments on the brain should follow clinical observations in order to confirm them; they are often misleading when they precede them.* All the motor and sensory centres will not explain the variety of mental powers, and the different degrees in which men are endowed with the same power. Motor and sensory centres will not explain why one vast intellect, like Newton's, fathoms the profundities of science, while the mind of another man scarcely gropes its way through the daily occurrences of life.

We all vary in our inborn mental dispositions, intellectual, emotional, and instinctive. If these dispositions depended on sensation alone, how could we explain why a particular impression leaves one man entirely unconcerned, inspires another to an artistic creation, fires a third to the deepest emotions, and rouses, in a fourth, some instinctive desires? It is not the external impressions that make the poet, musician, artist, philosopher, inventor; the humble and aggressive man; the timid and the brave man; the spendthrift and the avaricious man; the frank and the suspicious man. External impressions stimulate the innate disposition, but they do not create it. All the motor and sensory centres will not explain the difference between the constitution of the brain of a poetical genius, as compared, say, with a mathematical genius; or why a youth who, in all respects, is an idiot, should yet possess a remarkable memory for dates, or numbers, or localities, and be capable of practically all the emotions. Moreover, those who have observed the defective brains of idiots must be aware that they are often without any corresponding motor or sensory defect; and all the motor and sensory centres do not help us, even in the remotest way, to explain the facts of insanity. Some savage races have as much motor power and often more delicate senses than Europeans, and we ought to look to them for the most profound philosophy and the feeblest instincts. Persons blind, deaf, and dumb, from infancy—like that marvellous woman, Helen Keller—depending entirely on the sense of touch, are nevertheless capable of the highest intelligence and perfection of character.

The effect of the same sensation varies in each man according to his natural disposition; and, often, in the same man at different times. What sensation does is to rouse the mechanism of the brain centres for the primordial dispositions to activity, according to their relative development and associative arrangement. That is how the sight of, for example, a wood strikes the poet and timber merchant differently; and the hearing of the same sentence evokes different responses in different individuals.

No hypothesis of sensory brain centres will account for different persons being differently affected emotionally by the same news, received verbally or in writing; but, if it be admitted that the principal instincts and emotions have centres in the brain, then it can be easily understood that, according to the individual development of these centres, so will different people respond differently to the same stimulus.

It is not the perfection of the senses which gives intelligence to the brain, but the perfection of the brain which determines the employment of the senses. The senses are perfected in childhood, long before the structure of the brain is completed. The more primitive the brain organisation, as in the lower animals, the more will the response to sensations resemble reflex action; and the more organised the brain, the greater the control over the response.

Notwithstanding all the experiments on animal brains since the time of Rolando and Flourens, we have added but little to the knowledge possessed by the ancient Greeks—that we think with our brains. The fact that the environment stimulates that organ to respond with certain instinctive and emotional acts, has not yet been realised. That is to say, that besides observing, remembering, and reasoning, we also manifest love and hate, fear and courage, pride and modesty, cheerfulness and anger, through our brains. The experimenters on animals had failed to raise any such feelings at the point of their scalpel, and therefore they denied any relation between them and the brain.

The misleading nature of experiments on animals is proved by the fact that a slight blow to the human head may render a person insane; whereas, if we are to believe the experimenters, large portions of an animal's brain may be extirpated without affecting its mental condition. Physicians who attend to living humanity have observed that a slight injury to one part of the brain can affect a man's character and conduct in one particular manner, and leave him, in all other respects, a normal man. It will be shown in succeeding chapters that a blow to one particular region of the head may change the cheerful, optimistic man to a depressed and melancholic man, while injury of another part may cause a hitherto peaceful individual to become quarrelsome and violent, and a wound to another spot may cause a highly moral person to become a totally opposite character; and yet in all these cases, the intellect—that is to say, memory and reason—may remain quite unaffected. Consequently, I hold with Eugenio Tanzi (*Textbook of Mental Diseases*, 1909), that, "as the study of experimental localisation would appear to have reached its limit, *physiologists, in common with clinicians, and those who investigate the question from other standpoints, have now no reason to refuse space for a psychical zone*, the existence of which forces itself upon us, even apart from the testimony of experimental researches".

Charles Richet, twenty years earlier, was already sceptical. He then said (at the International Congress of Psychology in 1889): "Of course, we may disguise our ignorance under the imposing weight of fact, autopsy, or experiment. But, vulgarly speaking, this is merely throwing dust in our eyes; for the professor who cites the works of Ferrier, and of many other savants, must admit that our rich bibliography is but a delusive treasure; this abundance conceals profound poverty. The physiology of the brain is still shrouded in mystery. Cerebral physiology awaits some discovery of genius which will throw light on this problem, as mysterious to-day as it was two thousand years ago."

Now that experimental physiology has evidently done all it ever will do, towards elucidating the functions of the brain, any further advances must be made by observing the effect of injury and disease on man, since man is the only animal that can communicate his feelings, sensations, and thoughts by means of speech. In the human subject, strictly limited traumatic brain lesions are among the pathological conditions which bear most closely upon the problem of cerebral localisation. Necessarily, these accidental experiments upon the human brain are sometimes as sharply localised as are the experiments of the physiologist upon the brains of lower animals. For the purpose of the physician, indeed, they are more instructive than the latter; for they are not only limited in the area they involve—at all events at the time of the accident—but they are limited in the damage they do to the mentality of the victim. And, as I shall prove, whenever the same locality is affected, the same mental power undergoes a change. Similarly, circumscribed lesions, due to the growth of tumours, local haemorrhage, etc., give rise frequently to definite mental disturbances by the pressure they exert on a limited brain area. All these lesions may be described as Nature's own experiments, and, being made on man himself, are much more trustworthy and instructive than the experiments performed by physiologists on the lower animals. In fact, it is in cerebral pathology that we have the only sure means of control over physiological doctrines of the brain founded on experiment.

CHAPTER III

HISTOLOGICAL THEORIES

The part of the brain which is of importance to the manifestation of mental functions is the outer rind, or cortex, of grey matter, which is in contact with the inner surface of the skull. This outer rind is thrown into a series of tortuous folds or convolutions separated by slits or fissures, and both combine to give it an appearance of great complexity. These convolutions were long considered to present no definite arrangement, but to be thrown together in meaningless disorder. During the latter half, or rather more, of the last century, it has, however, been shown, by the many eminent men who have given their attention to the subject, that the pattern which is assumed by the convolutions—though showing many subsidiary differences, not only in different races and different individuals, but also in the two hemispheres of the same person—is yet arranged on a consistent and uniform plan in every human brain, and that any decided deviation from the plan results in an imperfect performance of the cerebral function.

The scholarly work of ALEXANDER ECKER on *The Convolutions of the Human Brain*, 1869, and that of GROMIER, entitled *A Study upon Cerebral Convolutions in Man and Monkey*, did much to lead men out of the labyrinth which draughtsmen represented very much as they would a dishful of macaroni. But if there is an orderly arrangement of the convolutions, the fact points to an orderly arrangement also in the psychical functions. This is the view taken by ECKER, in the work mentioned, when he wrote:

"That the cortex of the cerebrum, the undoubted material

substratum of our mental operations, is not a single organ, which is brought into play as a whole in the exercise of each and every psychical function, but consists rather of a multitude of organs, each of which is subservient to definite mental processes, is a conviction which forces itself upon us almost with the necessity of a claim of reason. The hypothesis, set up in opposition to it, of a single organ for carrying out the multiplicity of psychical functions, would present about an equivalent point of view to that of 'vital force', which has received its *coup de grâce. If, however, as we conceive to be an undoubted fact, certain portions of the cortex of the cerebrum subserve definite mental processes, the possibility is at once conceded that we shall some day arrive at a complete organography of the surface of the brain: a science of the localisation of the mental functions.* Such a science—that is, a knowledge of the psychological organs of the brain, in all their relations—is certainly one of the most important problems for the anatomy and physiology of the next century, the solution of which will work no small transformation in psychology."

So long as Flourens's theory of the unity of the brain prevailed, the microscopical structure of the different convolutions was regarded as uniform throughout; but, with the discovery of the speech centre, and, still more so, after the discovery of the motor centres, sixty years ago, interest in the minute anatomy of the brain was aroused; and this led to a new science—brain histology—with a host of eminent investigators: Purkinje, Lockhart Clarke, Bevan-Lewis, Meynert, Betz, Ramon-y-Cajal, Nissl, Golgi, Deiters, Donders, Weigert, Waldeyer, and others.

By the employment of refined histological methods it has been shown that the grey matter in the cortex of the hemispheres, and in other parts of the brain, is the seat of an enormous number of nerve cells, neurons, and that those in the cortex present many variations in form and size. Further, that these nerve cells give origin to axial nerve fibres, through which areas in the cortex become connected, directly or indirectly, either with other areas in the same hemisphere, or with parts at the base of the brain, and the spinal cord. Altogether, the microscopical study of the brain is now absorbing more attention than the naked-eye anatomy.

The neuron, the elementary unit of the nervous system, is formed of a nucleus and prolongations, which sometimes are of considerable length and differ morphologically and functionally in character. Some of these prolongations, possessing a structure closely resembling that of cellular protoplasm—the protoplasmic processes—are, generally speaking, numerous, relatively short, and ramify in the ganglionic mass in which the cell body lies. They subdivide, repeatedly, like the branches of a tree, and from this feature—forming arborisations—they are called dendrites. Another and thinner process—almost if not always single—is clearly seen to spring from the cell body, and splits up sooner or later into fine fibres, which in their turn may undergo further subdivision. This is the nerve process, neurite, axon, or axis-cylinder process. Although the neurons have one structural plan, and are all provided with a cell body, dendrites, and an axon, nevertheless, these organs differ immensely one from another in length, richness of ramifications, and in a thousand other morphological particulars.

It has been estimated, and held for a long time, that there are 9,200 millions of these neurons in the cerebral grey matter; but recently Prof. Constantin Economo, of Vienna, calculated that there are 14,000 millions of these cells.

Every neuron is anatomically quite distinct and separate from every other neuron. Yet the neuron cannot function alone, but must be linked up with others in conducting chains and arcs, and thus the impulse generated by any one neuron of necessity affects other neurons. Physiological contact between the neurons is established at the neuro-synapse, which is a short gap, a structural break, where the nervous impulse passes from one to the other, giving rise to the discharge of a fresh impulse. A stimulus to a nerve cell has been estimated to be capable of travelling to other cells at a speed of 125 metres a second.

Now, there are two schools of histologists. One, with by far the most numerous followers, attributes distinctive functions to the *horizontal* layers of the cortical cells. The nomenclature and interpretation varies somewhat with each observer, and so does the number of layers described.

J. Shaw Bolton distinguished five primary laminae, or layers of cells, in the cortex of the brain:

1. The outer fibre lamina or superficial layer.
2. The outer cell lamina or pyramidal layer.
3. The middle cell lamina or granule layer.
4. The inner fibre lamina.
5. The inner cell lamina or polymorphic layer.

Layers 1 and 2 were called by G. A. Watson: the supra-granular cortex; layer 3, the granular cortex; and layers 4 and 5, the infra-granular cortex.

The functions generally attributed by histologists to the various strata of cells are: "sensory", "perceptive", "association", "projection", "commemorative", and "psychical".

"Such and similar terms", said Brodmann (*Lokalisationslehre der Grosshirnrinde*, Leipsic, 1909), "which one meets on every step, especially in modern psychiatric and neurological literature, have no foundation; they are pure fiction, and serve no other purpose than to create confusion."

Carl Wernicke located in the most external layer "bodily consciousness"; in a deeper layer, "consciousness of the external world"; and in the lowest layer, that of "personality".

EMIL KRAEPELIN agreed with him.

According to Professor R. J. A. BERRY (*Brain and Mind*, New York, 1928), "the infra-granular cortex is largely concerned with animal reactions, on which the supra-granular cortex is partly inhibitory. If, therefore, the examination tends to show that the patient's brain is under-developed, it is a matter of practical certainty that it must be the supra-granular brain which is the more backward, and consequently the patient's reactions to the social environment will be more nearly on the animal plane of acquisition, and uncontrolled displays of sex."

We see, then, that histologists have tried to discover the different uses of the various layers of cells of the cortex of the brain; but unaided examination of structure has never yet been sufficient to reveal the functions of an organ. Even were we able to describe minutely the form of a cell, and the complicated network of the different granules which constitute it, we should not have got much further towards knowing its proper functions. The fact is, that dissection may prove the compatibility of function and structure, after the function is revealed by observation; or disprove an alleged function, by showing its incompatibility with well ascertained structure, We might dissect the optic nerve till the crack of doom, without being enabled, by that means alone, to demonstrate that its use is to convey visual impressions from the eye to the mind.

Whereas most histologists studied the layers of cortical cells in their *horizontal* aspect, another school, headed by BRODMANN, studied the *vertical* sections of the cortex and discovered that there are numerous groups, each of different structure and significance; indeed, that there occurs, throughout the mammalian series, in definite localities of the cortex, the same characteristic structural formation; so that homologous areas can be defined in the different animals, and in man, varying only in extent. This was confirmed by Professor G. Elliot Smith, who said (*Henderson Trust Lecture*, 1923):

"We know for certain that there is a very definite and precise anatomical localisation, i.e. *the cortex is divided up into a number of territories*, and presenting contrasts in appearance, of so marked type, that the boundary lines between these territories can be mapped out."

The cortex contains, according to these observers, a multiplicity of organs of different structural complexes, which we are led to assume, from the analogy of other organs, to have separate functions, so that the work hitherto performed by the whole brain is now split up and localised, the more precisely, the higher the animal in the scale of creation. Elliot Smith and Brodmann have made out about forty such structurally differentiated areas in the brain, as must exist, if localisation of mental functions is to be possible; but we are still left in ignorance of their functions. O. Vogt has since distinguished one hundred myelo-architectonic areas in the whole cortex, of which fifty are in the frontal lobes alone.

Considering Brodmann's discovery of so many anatomically distinguishable areas in the cortex, it is surprising to find that he is absolutely against the theory of localisation of mental functions; indeed, that he supports Flourens's contention that: "For every psychical action the whole brain is at work, and whatever psychical process is lost, is made up again by the remainder of the brain." However, he gives himself a loophole of escape from an otherwise untenable position by admitting the possibility that complex psychical states may be connected, as a "resultant", with certain definite areas, having—so to say—a "predilection" for them; but they are never the product of a morphological or physiological centre.

I fail to see that it matters whether certain complex psychical functions have a "predilection" for a "circumscribed" and "histologically distinct" part of the cortex, or whether they are the "resultant" of numerous minor processes all over the brain; or whether all the elements of a complex psychical function are to be found "associated" with that particular centre or organ. The "mind" may, or may not be, a product of the brain; but it is in some way associated with it; and the same can be said of its elements. What that relation really is, no one is yet in a position to say, but that need not hinder us from recording our observations of certain functions being abnormally performed, or inhibited, in certain definite lesions of the brain.

There are various institutes for Brain Research in existence all over the world: one, a famous one, in Leningrad, in Russia; one just opened in Berlin; and the Wistar Institute in Philadelphia, in the United States of America. Amongst other investigations, they conduct post-mortem examinations of the brains of eminent men. They measure and weigh these brains, and cut them up into microscopical slices; but nothing has so far been discovered to indicate what are the brain characteristics of men of genius. And no wonder; for the existing theories are all in a muddle. For instance, how can anatomists discover, in dissecting human brains, anything of the special structures involved in the different varieties of genius, when it is not even granted that the primary mental powers are at all localisable? If mental manifestation is dependent on brain structure and activity, it is full time we learnt something more about it than we know at present.

It seems, however, that the view is gaining ground that "special talents are due to differences in organisation of special parts of the cortex" (W. H. Howell, *A Textbook of Physiology*, 1918).

The most minute post-mortem examination of the brain structure under the magnifying lens can tell us nothing of the intellectual abilities, emotions, and passions of the living man. The brain of the Russian dictator, Lenin, who died some years ago, was cut, by Professor Vogt, into 31,000 microscopically minute sections; a feat in itself—but all in vain—for we do not yet know what to look for.

Enormous work has been done in recent years to discover changes in the brain cells in the various mental disorders. Histologists, like Shaw Bolton, have made important contributions to the pathology of amentia, dementia, and Sir Frederick Mott to dementia paralytica; but, as regards the general problem of the mental functions of the brain, and of insanity as a disease or disorder of the brain, we are still in the dark. Circumscribed lesions are rarely found in the brains of asylum patients. As a rule, either no change is found, for the want of a theory, when the particular disorder is declared to have been "functional"; or else the brain is vastly disorganised. It is only in cases when an intercurrent disease carries off the patient prematurely that one can expect post-mortem evidence of demonstrative value.

As far back as 1883, it was pointed out by Bevan-Lewis in which directions studies in cerebral localisation might advance our knowledge of insanity. He held that the localisation of cerebral function was the outcome of the great principle of evolution carried to its logical issue; that the alienist should rivet his attention upon the changes undergone by the material substrata of the mind; and he should, strictly and closely, study the objective manifestation of mental activity; *that he should learn to examine the various limited lesions of the cortex,* as to area, depth, localised atrophy, relative bulk of convolutions, and tracts of ascending and descending degeneration. This is quite true; but, without any theory of mental functions to guide us, we cannot learn much from it for the present.

Dr. Robert Hutchison contributed to the Edinburgh Hospital Reports, Vol. IV (reported in the *British Medical Journal,* 1896), a paper drawing attention to the fact that most asylum pathologists have too special an experience, and attribute all the changes found in patients dying in asylums to the insanity of which they died. He had taken the trouble to compare the histological appearances which are found in the brains of ordinary patients, dying in hospitals, with the changes found in the brains of the insane, and his conclusion was that, with the exception of general paralysis of the insane, very little that could be called special had been described by the asylum pathologist. Dr. Hutchison pointed out that, in other organs than the brain, a very large amount of disease or degeneration may be present, without interfering materially with the function of the organ, and he saw no reason why the brain—which certainly has a very large amount of surplus tissue—should not be able to work well, even though a good deal of local change in the cells had occurred. He considered that he had proved that similar changes occur, both in the brains of the sane and the insane; and he thought it would be hard to prove that the changes occur more frequently, and with greater intensity, in the insane than the sane.

Association Centres

There is still another localisation theory, that of the Association Centres, based on the fact that the brain fibres at the time of birth are not yet fully developed, and the various groups reach maturity (myelinisation) at different periods. This theory of association centres was founded by Professor Paul Flechsig, of Leipzig, some forty years ago, and, at the time, also led to great expectations which were not realised.

Flechsig distinguished four association centres:

1. The frontal brain proper;
2. A large portion of the temporal lobes;
3. A considerable area in the posterior parietal region;
4. The island of Reil.

We have, thus, four large and well-defined areas in the human brain which are not directly concerned with sensorial impressions from without and within, nor with motor impulses, but the activity of which is entirely directed inwards. These co-ordinating, or association centres, have received little support from clinical and experimental proof. Granted that such centres exist, they leave us still in the dark as to the origin of the primary mental powers, and the special abilities, with which man and animals are endowed. In my opinion the whole cortex of the brain consists of a mass of association centres. Thus Leonardo Bianchi, in his recent and most comprehensive work, *The Mechanism of the Brain and the Functions of the Frontal Lobes*, 1921, said:

"A problem of anatomy and psychology so important as this, considered without prejudice, cannot be solved solely by histological inquiries such as those of Flechsig, because it is proven that myelinisation of the endohemispheric fibres does not follow a constant law; and even if it did, it could not be inferred as a corollary without exception, that this geography of evolutionary anatomy should be regarded as a sure foundation for a species of psychological geography. If we follow the inductive method of reasoning, we are obliged to conclude that *myelinisation of the fibres leading to the so-called association centres has nothing to do with the evolution of intelligence*, for the simple reason that, whilst the fibres of the terminal territories are developed in the fourth, and often as late as the tenth month after birth, intelligence is not developed until a much later period. *There is no correspondence between the development of mental phenomena and that of the anatomical territories assigned to them.* The histological factor, as Brodmann has remarked, remains to some extent detached from the psychological factor, and does not offer a satisfactory explanation of the latter."

It is evident that the microscopical study of brain cells has so far not succeeded in disclosing the relation between mind and brain. I am only stating facts as I see them, and by no means under-estimate the splendid work done by histologists. The fault is in the method, and what we expect from it. Does anyone really anticipate that even the most scrupulous examination of a brain cell will ever reveal the thought or feeling of a living man? What is there to show the anatomist who is dissecting the brain, or holding a section under the microscope, that a particular group of brain cells is agitated in love, fear, or anger; or invoked in the production of a sentiment in the exercise of logic?

Is insanity due to cerebral disorder? If this question were put to psychiatrists, the answer we should receive would be unanimously "Yes!" Yet, if we look into textbooks on Insanity, for confirmation of this statement, we shall find that, with the exception of such destructive diseases as General Paralysis and Chronic Dementia, there is no proof at all that the greater number of recognised mental disorders derange the brain even in the slightest degree; on the contrary, they are described, most of them, as if they were purely psychical. The reason for this omission is that we know nothing definite of the mental functions of the brain, and that, consequently, the pathologist is at a loss what to look for. The plain fact is that too much has been made of the experimental and histological investigations into the functions of the brain. I am not deriding them; I am only trying to assign them to their proper place. All I want is to protest against the exaggerated estimation of laboratory work, by which all those who are engaged in it, and who explain the mysteries of life and disease by physical, mechanical, and chemical laws, are hailed as scientists, and none others are considered to deserve the name, or merit serious attention.

CHAPTER IV

THE NEGLECT OF SYSTEMATIC CLINICAL OBSERVATION

We have seen that physiologists recognise only motor and sensory centres; but it is evident that, behind these centres, there lie also all the functions which constitute mental phenomena. It has also been shown that the study of the microscopical appearance of the brain has produced magnificent results, but has failed, so far, to explain the nature of mental activities and disorders of the mind. Chemical and glandular theories, too, have thrown some light on the special mental disorders which are caused by such agencies, but do not touch the great problems concerning mind and brain. Insanity will never be explained until we admit that the primary psychical activities are dependent on definite and separate instruments. In my opinion, *it is because of the non-recognition of the principle of localisation of mental functions that so little progress has been made, both in the study and treatment of brain disease and mental disorder.* Most insanities, as I have pointed out, are held to be purely functional, and others are assumed to involve the entire brain; consequently, clinical observation is believed to be of little practical use, even where opportunities are given.

Every decided advance in the knowledge of the localisation of functions has been due to the careful collation and comparison of cases with autopsies and the study of their common features. It is by the observation of clinical and pathological data, chiefly, that we can hope to discover the mental functions of the brain and their localisation. Clinical experience is, after all, the most important, and it has already taught us a good deal.

Post-mortem investigations alone, without a study of the patient while alive, are unsatisfactory; for the disease, in persons who have died insane, has converted the edifice of the mind into a mass of ruins. This puts the pathologist almost in the same position as a man would be who were to inspect fireworks on the morning after the display is over. The living phenomena are gone, and, with them, the key to the explanation of the structural changes. Nor can the bacteriologist, or physiological chemist, explain the working of the human mind independently of the physician. The things they have found are discoveries of great importance; but they explain only the proximate, and not the essential, cause of insanity. They are the sparks, as it were, which ignite the fireworks. A knowledge of the igniting impulse, and a study of the remains of the fireworks, are extremely useful; but they do not explain the combustion. For this purpose we must actually witness the display, and this is done by the physician who attends and treats the living patient.

The alienists, whose proper department is mind and its disorders, have rarely the opportunity of collecting such material. They attend to the living patient, but, as I have already said, unless he dies of an intercurrent disease, the brain does not come under observation until it is severely disorganised by advanced dementia. Besides, not all asylums or mental hospitals are fitted with pathological laboratories.

The asylums for the insane admit only advanced and, more or less, chronic cases. Moreover, they are like monasteries of the past, on beautiful heights in the country, surrounded by big walls, which not only prevent the escape of patients, but by the rules with which these institutions are governed, prevent anyone but its salaried officers making clinical studies within them. We try to learn the mind and character of man, and the structure and functions of the brain, from the results of the irritation and mutilation of animals; but the vast material always at our disposal, in the large number of asylums all over the world, is barred, even to expert physicians. If they were thrown open to a visiting staff, as hospitals are, we should be enabled to examine the mentality of our patients in a systematic manner, and, after death, view their brains both macroscopically and microscopically. Moreover, asylum officers are burdened with so many administrative duties, that only those who really love their work, and are born with a gift for it, ever make any contributions to our knowledge of the subject.

No wonder that, until a few years back, it was frequently denied that there is any difference between the brains of sane and insane; and now, when we have a fair number of pathological laboratories connected with asylums, the only definite facts we possess are, as has been pointed out, the appearance of brains in amentia and dementia (progressive, alcoholic, and senile). It is to be borne in mind that even when the patient dies early, no circumscribed lesion may be discovered; for, without a localisation theory, the pathologist is obliged to take, at random, slices from any part of the brain. However carefully and minutely he may examine the microscopical appearance of these sections, his descriptions, though valuable from other points of view, will not help us in the solution of this most important problem.

We rarely get clinical cases, with post-mortem observations, reported from asylums, except by those who study histological changes. The few *mental* cases which are recorded in medical periodicals are by neurologists and surgeons.

Experiments on animals can produce only motor and sensory phenomena. Therefore, physiologists lay stress on them, and, clinical observation not coming within their range, they are apt to undervalue it in comparison with their own more exact research. But now that experimental physiology of this kind has practically been given up, any further advance, I emphasise once more, must be made by observing the effects of injury and circumscribed disease on the human subject.

Often it is only some local irritant to the membranes of the brain which causes the mental changes—such as a splinter of bone, accumulation of fluid, etc.—while the general brain condition remains perfectly sound. In such cases, cranial operation is all that is needed for the relief of the patient; and the more alarming brain surgery need not be undertaken. From the cases quoted in the succeeding chapters, it will be seen that there is no apparent limit to the time that may elapse before surgical treatment may be carried out successfully. Some of the cases have been treated three, four, eight, and eleven years after the accident; one case even after twenty-five years.

Similarly, circumscribed lesions due to the growth of tumours, local haemorrhage, etc., give rise frequently to definite mental symptoms by pressure on a specific brain area. But such clinical observations are rarely made systematically. Neurologists observe principally visual, auditory, and speech phenomena, but with reference to mind proper—as including intellectual capacities, emotions, and instincts—these are rarely noted by them, and changes so severe as to amount to insanity do not come within their sphere.

Let us take, for example, a big work like that by H. Duret, *Les Tumeurs de l'Encéphale*, Paris, 1915. It contains the records of not less than 399 cases of brain tumours, mentioning every variety of neurological symptoms; but no mental changes, except in one or two cases, in which it is recorded, in a vague way, that there were "troubles psychiques".

At a joint meeting of the Sections of Neurology and Psychiatry at the Royal Society of Medicine on February 12th, this year, a discussion took place on "Mental Symptoms associated with Brain Tumours", when the chairman, Dr. Kinnier Wilson, in summing up, said that "all neurologists appeared to agree that the localising value of mental symptoms in cerebral tumour was relatively *nil*".

It is not uncommon to find patients some years after the occurrence of a head injury present symptoms of mental deterioration due to degenerative changes set up in the cortical layers of the hemispheres. The mischief produced may be out of all proportion to the apparent severity of the lesion, and, therefore, such injury should never be lightly regarded. The instructive matter in these cases is that the moral character is usually impaired first, and is sometimes completely perverted without a corresponding deterioration of the understanding. Yet we still find physicians and surgeons who neglect to inquire into the condition of the emotions and propensities, in brain lesions, and proceed as if the human mind consisted of intellect only. This lack of appreciation of the character changes, following upon circumscribed injury or disease, need not surprise us, for insanity has not long been recognised as a morbid condition of the brain, and it is only about eighty years ago that the Royal College of Physicians of London published a *Nomenclature of Diseases*, in which insanity was dissociated from all other affections which beset humanity, and its varieties were comprised under the heading "Disorders of the Intellect"—all connection with the emotions and instinctive dispositions being denied.

It is due to a lack of proper psychological training and

inadequate knowledge of the elements of human character that the statement is so frequently made that "all the faculties have been found entire" after a brain lesion. If a man were reduced mentally by disease to the state of a dog, or idiot, he would still possess the general faculties of perception, memory, and judgment; at all events in ordinary affairs, and it might be said all his faculties remained entire. For example, the most incredible case ever quoted is a recent one, by WALTER DENBY (*Journal of American Medical Association*, 1928), who had removed the *entire right hemisphere* in an operation. The patient, who actually lived three and a half years longer, is claimed by Dr. Denby not to have suffered any marked mental impairment.

The mental examination of patients with brain lesions will have to be conducted on very different lines in the future, if we are to make any progress with the discovery of the mental functions of the brain. Every structure in the nervous system has a specified function, and, if a portion is destroyed, it cannot be replaced anatomically; and, further, from the point of view of function, the compensations which are provided indirectly are always far from being complete. If, in such cases, no defect is recognised, it must undoubtedly be due to insufficient methods, to which may be added, perhaps, a want of patience on the part of the observer.

Possibly instances of extensive cerebral disorganisation do occur, in which neither mental, nor motor, nor sensory disturbances appeared during life, of so marked a character as to excite a suspicion that such things existed; but this kind of anomaly is by no means limited to the brain. Numerous cases are recorded in which a whole lung has been destroyed, or the greater part of the liver disorganised, or a kidney has disappeared, without any suspicion having been entertained during life of the real state of matters; and it would obviously be as reasonable to infer from them that the lungs were not the organs of respiration, or the liver not the organ of secretion of bile.

As there is no definite method followed in observing character changes, we get such statements as that "Abscess of the brain may exist, or portions of the brain be carried away by gunshot or other injuries, and yet no perceptible difference be observed in the mentality of the individual". After reading this, one wonders what really is the use of the brain. It is only the vague, indefinite manner in which all these examples are produced that saves the head and its contents from the imputation of being useless appendages. The brain is the instrument of all the mental powers, and it betrays great indifference to assert that it matters not whether the instrument be a whole or a broken one.

That lesions of the brain may be the actual and direct cause of mental derangement, can scarcely be doubted. In certain cases, in which there has been gross lesion of the brain or its membranes, and in which insanity has developed immediately, or later, in connection with certain symptoms dating from the injury, we are justified in concluding that there is a direct causal relation. This view is strongly supported by the fact that complete and prompt recovery has followed surgical operation in many cases of this nature.

A fact that is frequently overlooked is that the brain is composed of two similar halves, or hemispheres, and that, consequently, all the centres are double. The wonder is that one-sided injury so often causes loss of a particular mental power, at least in the frontal lobes; for one would expect it to be necessary for both centres to be destroyed to cause the functions with which it is connected to disappear.

Another difficulty is the fact that the site of the injury does not always give a correct idea of the area of the brain that has been damaged. The lesion may extend downwards, and disrupt the connecting fibres to other centres, which thus get involved. Such a condition cannot be discovered during the lifetime of the patient. It can only be surmised by the symptoms presented.

Still another difficulty is that none of the brain areas possessing special functions are of definite outline, and may therefore present complex symptoms of more than one region. Considering there are so few mental cases reported in our medical journals, it is wonderful that I have found them—with few exceptions—when proper details were given, to substantiate the localisations given in this book.

There must be a division of labour in the cortex, as elsewhere; and certain groups of cells will be occupied more readily with one fundamental quality, rather than with another. But that does not say that destruction of a particular area of the brain, even if we know its exact boundaries, need necessarily cause loss of a definite mental function, for no centre ever works alone; just as we can rarely think of one subject or event, without being reminded of a number of others, associated with it, and having various feelings aroused at the same time.

Though the brain centres themselves are distinct, all of them are inter-united; and the activity of each depends on its relation to the others. None of the centres can be completely disjointed. Each of them acts as a certain portion of the brain, to modify the general result of cerebral action. The different centres are only points of highest activity of a special function, and each specialised group of cells is connected with a number of other groups. Consequently, when one centre is roused into activity, the greater part, if not the whole, of the brain may react in unison. All the centres may, therefore, be regarded as association or co-ordinating centres. It is through this solidarity and inter-dependence that no portion of the brain can be injured, or exhausted, without its interfering, in some way, with the functions of the other portions. *There is, however, a great difference between saying that the various brain parts exert a mutual influence, and saying that each part does not perform its own particular function.*

In 1884, in his dispute with Munk and Goltz, HITZIG wrote as follows: "I adhere to-day to the hypothesis I put forward in 1870, that the *cortical centres are merely collecting centres.* I can support the opinion, which has often been expressed, that *deep or very extensive lesions, affecting the central mechanism, necessarily interrupt a multitude of bundles* which unite different cortical regions of the brain with one another, and must, consequently, give rise to symptoms that are susceptible to a relatively rapid improvement.

It has also to be noted that diagnosis, in cases of blows to the head, is often rendered difficult because of the effects of *contre-coup*. The head may be struck on the occiput, but the concussion causes the brain to shoot forward and impinge upon the frontal bone, where the effects may be produced. Were the mental functions of the brain better known, we should be more certain when a *contre-coup* has taken place, and would not have to wait for the post-mortem examination.

Another, and avoidable, circumstance leading to errors in localising lesions, arises from the fact that so few physicians are intimately acquainted with the relation of the convolutions to the skull bones. To mention only one instance. I have found critics of my localisations unaware of the extent of the posterior part of the frontal lobes. Symptoms which I have ascribed to them, they show to have been in the superior parietal area, because the superior part of the parietal bone was injured. Now, the fissure of Rolando, which divides the frontal lobe from the parietal lobe in each hemisphere, is situated at a variable distance behind the coronal suture. "The more highly developed the frontal lobe of the brain is, the more oblique is the fissure of Rolando", according to ECKER (*Convolutions of the Human Brain*). Sir WILLIAM TURNER, among other anatomists, found its upper extremity sometimes as much as two inches behind the top of the suture joining the frontal and parietal bones; and its lower end as much as an inch and a half behind the lower extremity of the same. Not only the frontal, but also the parietal, temporo-sphenoidal and occipital lobes, take their names after the cranial bones; but these lobes are not wholly situated within the boundaries of the respective bones from which they derive their names. Often the very men who claim to have disproved my theory, unknowingly quote cases of their own which actually confirm it. (See examples in Chapters VI and VII.)

I have shown in the previous chapter that the views on localisation are very conflicting. Consequently, the wisest plan for physicians and surgeons to follow would be to content themselves with placing on record the facts they observe, and let them, as it were, speak for themselves. If, as hitherto, every observer has his own preconceived notions, and draws conclusions from one or two cases that have come under his care, his report is useless; just as much as is the report of that other man whose mind is "made up" that localisation of any sort is impossible.

Thus, many surgeons hold that injuries to the head do

not affect the mental powers; while other surgeons describe a "traumatic insanity", as if the symptoms were always the same, no matter what region of the head is injured. Most observers think the matter of so little importance that they give a very vague description of the locality of the lesion. We find such statements as "patient received a blow on the head", or, "there was a scar on the side of the head", without telling us what bone had been injured, and what part of it.

Surgeons are not really the best judges of the problem before us, for they are generally in a hurry, necessarily so, and have no time, even if they have the opportunity, to make detailed examination of the patient's mentality, or to follow up the case. Thousands of operations have been performed, in the recent war, for injuries to the skull and brain, and, as in olden times, so now, the statement is made in the medical reports that the patient suffered neither in intellect nor character, though he lost an appreciable quantity of brain matter. The surgeon may be right; but he should state what sort of examination he made into the mental condition of the patient, and *how long after the operation he had him under observation.*

It has been my experience that, whenever a patient is able to return a rational answer to any simple question about his health, the surgeon and attendants invariably speak of him as in full possession of all his faculties. So long as the patient can answer ordinary questions about his food, number of his family, his location at the time, and attend to his bodily wants with some care, he is considered not to have shown any mental symptoms. But I have had the opportunity of following-up several of these cases, and have discovered, not only some with loss of definite intellectual capacities, and certainly diminished vigour of the mental powers; but, in a great many instances, marked emotional changes—from previous cheerfulness to melancholy, from gentle peacefulness to irascibility, from affection to hatred, from honesty and truthfulness to deceitfulness and criminal tendencies. Are these changes of character and conduct not also due to the brain lesions? I am in a position to affirm that, if such changes were taken notice of at the time, or the possibility of their later development recognised, measures might be taken, which, in many cases, would save a man from the workhouse, prison, or asylum. The man with a serious brain injury has few needs, few thoughts, few feelings, and is only semi-conscious for some time after the accident; the questions usually put to him convey no information about his real state, and allow no estimate of his future conduct. Let us follow up the history of such cases, after the patients have returned to ordinary life; and a different picture will be presented. They are not the men they were before.

A man may give correct answers to questions put to him at the bedside of a general hospital, and yet be totally changed in character, since his illness commenced. Even a common cold can lower the mental energy and cause irritability; and yet a severe gunshot injury is sometimes stated to have made no difference to the patient's mental capacity. Indeed, unless a man becomes so demented as to neglect the ordinary wants of nature, or so furious, maniacal, or irrational as to require restraint, there are few surgeons who inquire narrowly into a patient's mental state.

Those who do not expect to find localised areas of disease in mental derangement, are not looking for them. To them, it matters nothing whether a person be melancholic, violently maniacal, homicidal, or suffering from delusions of persecution; whether he be a kleptomaniac, religious maniac, or self-styled millionaire, they assume in every case that the whole brain is affected. But, if we are disputing one of the most elementary problems of the functions of the brain, what advances can be made in the treatment of the insane and feeble-minded?

The current opinion appears to be that all abnormal mental manifestations are purely *functional*. This is the view expressed as recently as September 18th, 1926, in the *British Medical Journal*, in reply to an inquiry for "the best and latest work on Insanity as showing that insanity and other abnormal mental conditions are due to structural alterations in the brain caused by disease or injury or other defect". This was the answer:

"That insanity and other abnormal mental conditions are due to *structural* alterations in the brain is a thesis now seldom advanced in psychiatric textbooks. The proposition as it stands, is, in our present state of knowledge, unproven. Most observers, however, firmly believe that in all such conditions there is some functional disorder of the brain, presumably of a biochemical nature; and that there may, of course, be simultaneous functional derangements of the endocrine organs and the vegetative nervous system, which are possibly causative."

Owing to these views, the number of observations really available for scientific purposes is comparatively small. If the records of these cases were more carefully taken—both as regards the extent and location of the injury, as well as to the mental changes following it—we should obtain most valuable information; whereas now this vast material is almost lost to us.

I do not claim that all the cases quoted by me are perfect;

possibly some may be objected to on closer inquiry. But, whatever the defect of the individual cases, I hope I have produced such a volume of evidence as shall induce—not necessarily the acceptance of my theories—but a *fresh investigation into the whole subject of mental functions*, on the lines suggested by me. And, of course, not on the basis of former cases, but on new ones, as they happen to occur.

It may be objected that many of the cases cited by me are not recent ones; some might even be described as ancient. But is this really a vital objection to the theories advanced? Such facts as our modern students being trained to devote all their attention to the microscopical appearances of the brain in the different psychoses, to the neglect of naked-eye appearances; the prevalence of endocrine and toxin theories—and of recent years of psychological theories—to account for most forms of insanity; the lack of opportunity to study the early stages of mental disorders; the fact that intellectual changes are not inquired into with sufficient minuteness, and character changes are often disregarded altogether; the surgical cases not being observed long enough; and last, but not least, the contempt with which the localisation theory of *mental* functions has hitherto been regarded, explain sufficiently the lack of adequate material.

A puzzling difficulty to some observers is that in lesions of the brain the particular mental function is sometimes manifested more intensely; at other times it is diminished, or lost. This is explained by the inflammation preceding the destruction of the nerve cell. During the process of inflammation, the activity of the function connected with the area involved will be stimulated to hyperactivity; and when degeneration commences, and destruction takes place, the function connected with the circumscribed area will diminish or vanish. This is in agreement with the law of the "temporary excess of function in atrophy", by Claude Bernard, which is that: "When a histological element dies, or tends to die, its irritability, before diminishing, begins to augment, and it is only after this exaltation that it decreases again, and gradually becomes extinct." It has also to be noted that, when the region of the intellectual functions is damaged, these become lost; but when the region of the emotions and propensities is injured, these become augmented. As a rule, the emotions become accentuated in inflammatory lesions of the parts of the brain concerned with them, while intellectual powers appear to be lost. (For proof of this statement see Chapters VI, VII, and VIII.)

We must distinguish between irritative and destructive lesions; the one augments the activity, the other destroys the mental power. Irritation of the frontal lobes, for example, causes flight of ideas, remarkable memory for facts and events, quick reasoning, and so on; their destruction is followed by apathy, slow mental responses, and lack of attention and interest.

This question of localisation of function is of the highest importance, both to the psychologist and the physician. The localisation theory will enable us to explain abnormalities of character, and to trace them to their cause; and will help us in the diagnosis and treatment of the early stages of mental derangement.

As Charles K. Mills, Professor of Neurology in the University of Pennsylvania, has said:

"In some quarters a tendency to rebel against the extreme differentiation of the brain into areas and sub-areas and centres is exhibited; but close attention to the facts—particularly those which are being obtained through clinico-pathological observation—would seem to show that this differentiation is even much greater than has been supposed by the most ardent believer in localisation. . . . If the insanities are essentially disorders of the brain—as all must admit in a final analysis of the subject—and if the brain is recognised—not as an organ all parts of which are necessary to every function, or an organ one part of which is sufficient for all functions, but as an assemblage or confederation of separate organs, or centres, each of which is independent, or, at least, autonomous, it follows that the facts and principles of cerebral localisation must play an important rôle in the solution of psychiatric problems, and, especially, in the elucidation of psychic symptoms, and the causation, duration, and the prognosis, of the different types of insanity."

We are brought thus to realise that relation between mental activities and brain functions is a highly intricate problem of the utmost importance. Undoubtedly, the old methods of research have failed to disclose mental functions. The sooner, therefore, we can find new methods to solve this problem, the better it will be for medical science and humanity.

Thirty years ago I advanced the theory that lesions of the frontal lobes give rise to cheerfulness and self-satisfaction; lesions of the central and posterior parietal regions, to self-depreciation, depression, and, not infrequently, to a tendency to suicide; and lesions of the lower part of the temporal lobes, to states of irritation, anger, violence, and, occasionally, to a tendency to homicide. I shall give, in later chapters, a vast collection of cases confirming this theory; but will mention here only three typical cases of brain tumours as an example.

Case of Frontal Tumour with Cheerfulness.

THOMAS LYLE (*Journal of Mental Science*, 1880):

T. H., a boatman, "keeps in the very best of spirits. When asked how he is, says he feels 'very well', repeating the words 'very well'. He sings occasionally, and talks a good deal of the fine boats he possesses, and addresses strangers by some familiar name, such as 'Joe'; labours under the delusion of mistaken identity, and holds out his hand to shake hands with strangers, believing he has known them all his life. Takes his food well, and enjoys it. *Generally very happy and contented.*" Post-mortem, a tumour was found occupying the greater part of the right frontal lobe.

Case of Parietal Tumour with Apprehension, Mental Depression, and Suicidal Tendency.

C. v. Monakow (*Archiv. f. Psychiatrie*, 1881):

R., a well-to-do farmer's wife, age fifty-three, had no illness until her fortieth year, when she became melancholic, with intense depression and self-accusations. Six years in the asylum. Seven years later relapse with morbid fears and suicidal tendency. Re-admitted. Her anxiety much worse, hardly any sound sleep, *wept and wailed for days together*, accused herself of impiety, and deemed this the cause of her illness. *Intellect unclouded*, no hallucinations. She died after five years. The autopsy revealed two sarcomatous tumours in the left parietal lobe, which had grown together and had perforated the bone. They involved the gyri supra-marginalis and angularis and surrounding brain substance.

Case of Temporal Tumour with Irascibility.

William Boyd and Stanley Hopwood (*Lancet*, 1913):

A man, age forty-seven, by trade a moulder, suffering from chronic mania, a useful and capable worker in the asylum, though weak-minded, and having auditory hallucinations. He had *periodic attacks of noisy excitement, and at times became very abusive.* He died after ten years' residence. Post-mortem, the greater part of the left temporal lobe was replaced by a large cyst. Remainder of brain normal.

PLATE IV

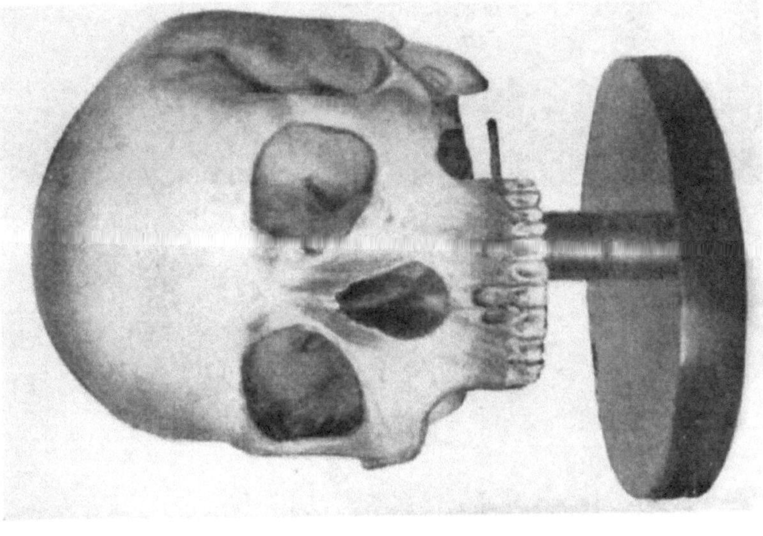

MODERN EUROPEAN SKULL

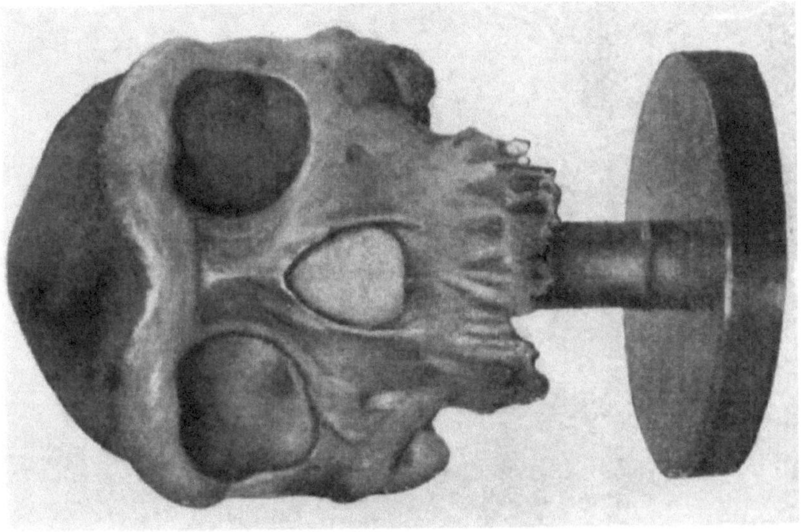

PREHISTORIC SKULL FOUND AT BROKEN HILL IN RHODESIA (1920)

(*See page* 263)

PLATE V

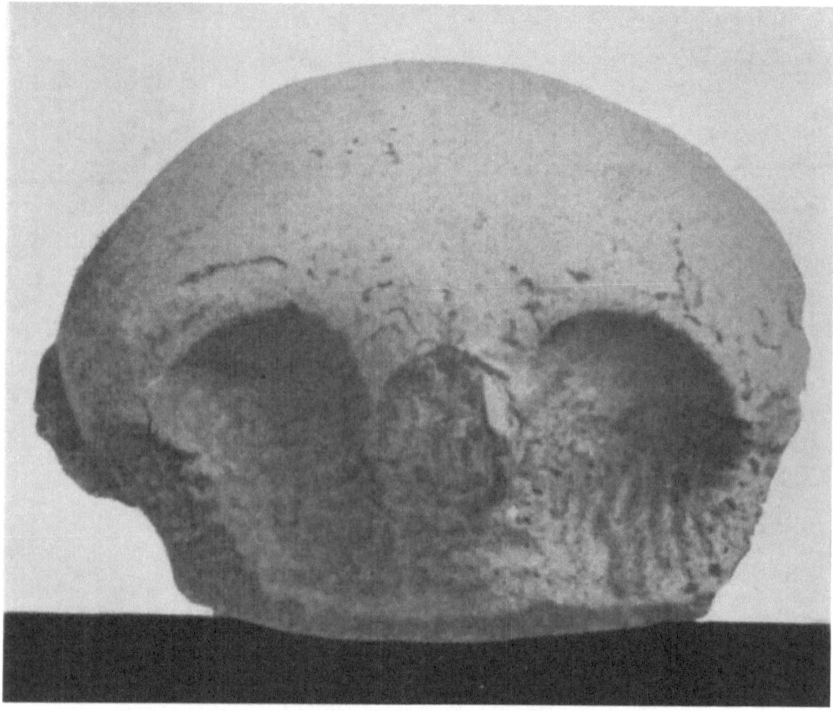

PREHISTORIC SKULL (GIBRALTAR)

Recently discovered. Estimated 20,000 years old (*see page* 263)

CHAPTER V

IS SIZE OR WEIGHT OF BRAIN A MEASURE OF INTELLIGENCE?

Other things being equal, the greatest amount of mental capacity and vigour is allied with the largest quantum of cerebral substance. All observation, as regards men and animals, proves that the energy of any nervous centre always bears a direct proportion to its bulk, whether absolute or relative. Every organ of our body increases in size, in proportion to its exercise, within the limits of its physiological capacity, and this holds good with regard to the brain. With increased mental work, the brain will show an increased growth.

AMADEI, MEYNERT, SOMMER, and PELI, claimed that their measurements showed the *cranial capacity* to be greater in the insane (presumably in the active forms of insanity) than the sane; the constant mental exercise increasing the size of their brain. The tables of the *weights* of the brain in the insane which have been published by BOYD, PARCHAPPE, and THURNAM, furnish many examples of brains which weighed 55 oz. and upwards. The greatest weights are those of people having suffered from mania.

The size of the entire head shows the mental power only; not the mental correctness. The town clock may operate with a degree of power in proportion to its size, and may be heard resounding throughout a whole city, exercising, thereby, a widespread influence; and yet a small watch may excel it in point of correctness. Likewise, a little man with a small head may excel, in correctness, a big man with a large head, by reason of a more perfect proportion of the several parts of the brain and a better cultivation of his mental powers.

Mere size of brain indicates brain power only—as a large boiler will generate more steam than a small one—*but does not indicate its direction, whether in intellect, emotional feeling, or animal passion.* A man, like an animal, may have a large mass of brain, and yet not manifest much intelligence; but both will exhibit power of some sort or other.

The average circumference of the head is 22½ in. in males and 21½ in. in females; and the longitudinal measurement, from the root of the nose over the crown of the head to the occipital protuberance, is on an average 14 in. Measures much below this point to some degree of mental deficiency.

The average cubic capacity of the skull, according to MANOUVRIER, is 1,560 cubic centimetres in ordinary men, and 1,665 c.c. in eminent men; and, according to BORDIER, 1,540 c.c. in murderers.

The average length of skull is 190 mm. (7·48 in.). The highest point of the vault reaches 100 mm. above the base, i.e. above the sub-cerebral plane.

Heads measuring 11 to 13 inches in circumference, and with a longitudinal diameter—from the glabella (root of the nose) to the occipital spine—of 8 to 9 inches, belong to the lowest class of idiots, in whom the intellectual manifestations are nil.

If we find a circumference of 14 to 17 inches, and a longitudinal measurement of 11 to 12 inches, in an otherwise well-proportioned head, we may expect so small a size to be accompanied by a proportionate degree of stupidity or fatuity, combined, more or less, with inability to fix the attention upon a determinate object. In addition, we shall discover vague sentiments, indeterminate and transitory affections and passions, an irregular train of ideas; speech consisting of broken phrases, or merely of substantives or verbs—as to eat, to walk, to play, etc.; blind and irregular instincts, or an almost entire absence of them.

Heads of 18 or 18½ inches in circumference are small, yet if well-balanced, they are not incompatible with the regular exercise of the intellectual powers. They indicate, however, a pitiful mediocrity; a slavish spirit of imitation; credulity; superstition; that species of sensibility which by a trifle is raised to the height of joy, or plunged into an abyss of tears; a very fallible judgment; an extreme difficulty in discerning the relation of cause and effect; a want of self-control; and, frequently—which is a happy circumstance—but few desires. With this degree of development, however, there may exist some marked mental aptitudes—such as a remarkable memory for figures, dates, music, etc., because some cerebral part may be more fully developed.

As a rule, however, when the brain is too small, it is not dwarfed equally, in all its parts, but is specially so in the pre-frontal and frontal regions—in those parts which, as will be shown, manifest the peculiarly human faculties and sentiments; while the hinder and lower parts of the brain—those which appear to be the seats of the propensities—are far less affected; hence, also, the peculiarly animal look.

Absolute size is not a measure of development, because the brain must bear a certain relationship to the size of the body, in all classes of animals. Consequently, a very large animal of a lower class will necessarily have a larger brain than a very small animal of a higher class. For example, the brain of a large shark is very small, compared with the size of the animal; but it is much larger, absolutely, than the brain of a mouse, which, though absolutely small, presents evidences of a higher development than the other. We cannot, then, from the mere size or weight of the brain in any given case, arrive at a just conclusion regarding the state of development of the organ. Among animals of the same kind, the absolute size of the brain may lead to conclusions regarding the weakness or strength of their cerebral *power*; but no conclusion can be drawn, from absolute size alone, as to the mental *capacities* of the animal.

On the other hand, the relative size of the brain to that of the whole body of the animal is not a measure of the mental capacity either. In general, as animals rise in the scale, so their brains become, not only more complex, but larger in proportion to the size of the whole body. But, although this observation applies to the great majority of animals, still, the exceptions are numerous, and the laws of nature have no exceptions.

While the weight of the brain is somewhat proportionate to the weight of the body, the relative weight of the brain and body varies markedly among different animals. The relative size of the brain is greater among smaller animals. The elephant and whale have proportionately smaller brains than man; and the song-birds, apes, and mice, proportionately larger brains than man. The brain of the canary, and many other birds, constitutes a twenty-fifth part of their whole weight; whereas the brain of the elephant—in every respect more fully developed than that of birds—does not weigh a thousandth part of the huge body of the animal. So that we may not conclude that even the relatively larger brains indicate greater degrees of intelligence. It has been shown, however, that if one compares the weight of the brain and spinal cord, the weight of the brain of man is greater, in proportion to the spinal cord, than that of any other mammal. In man, the weight of the cord is about 2 per cent. of the brain weight; in apes about 6 per cent.; and ranges from 23 to 47 per cent. among other mammals.

Moreover, the body varies at different periods of life; whereas the brain undergoes no corresponding change. Besides, small heads are often found in big men, and large heads in short, light-weighted men. The relative size of the brain, then, to the whole body, cannot be viewed as a test or measure of cerebral development.

Mere size of a brain conveys nothing, without a knowledge of the quality of its texture. A large head may yet lack depth of convolution, and possess an inadequate number of brain cells. But we have yet to learn what is a normal brain, in this respect. Most of the brains that have been studied, so far, have been of men dying in pauper institutions or in hospitals; that is, brains affected by senile changes, degenerative processes, or active disease.

As a rule, all the parts of the same brain have the same quality. But, if we compare two brains, we must recollect that their size may be equal, and that, nevertheless, the one, through possessing the finer texture, and its owner having a more vigorous bodily constitution, may be active and energetic; while the other, being inferior in quality, or its owner of a different temperament, or feebler constitution, is naturally inert.

Even when the size, shape, and quality of the brain prove favourable, it is not certain that the mental operations will be well performed; for there are still other things which might impart unusual energy, or impede the activity of the brain. The digestion, circulation, or other function, may be out of order, and exert an exciting or deteriorating influence on the brain, however well proportioned; besides, the amount and consistency of the internal glandular secretions may have an accelerating or retarding effect on the cerebral functions.

It is evident, also, that if the mental functions of the brain include emotional and instinctive activities, as well as intellectual, *we must not confuse the two terms, "mental" and "intellectual"*. The former means the whole mind: feeling, thinking, acting; but the latter means, or refers to, only one of the three divisions of mind, namely, the thinking property. Now, the word mental, as applied to its organ, embraces the entire brain; but the word intellectual, when used to designate its organ, merely refers to, or embraces, the part of the brain to which the intellect is more especially related, namely, according to our theory, the frontal lobes. *Size and weight of the whole brain, are, therefore, not measures of the intellectual capacity of a man, but of his mind, his mental power—without determining whether that power lies in extent of intellect, in strength of moral feeling, or in force of passion, or affection.* Through ignorance of this fact the objection arose, that, while some men had large heads, other men of eminence have had small ones.

On a rough estimation, the size of the purely intellectual region ranges from about one-fourth to about one-third of the whole brain. Hence, a man with great intellect combined with little sentiment and passion, might have a small brain and, consequently, a small head; while, on the other hand, a man of strong passions, great impulsive energy, and strong sentiment, will have a large head, whether his intellect be strong or feeble. A big-headed man may manifest considerable mental power in the feelings and passions, and but little in the direction of the intellect; while a small-headed man may be all intellect.

From this it follows that the practice of measuring the size and weight of the entire brain, or of measuring the circumference of skulls, or calculating the cephalic index: $\frac{\text{breadth of skull} \times 100}{\text{length}}$—on which so much reliance is placed

PLATE VI

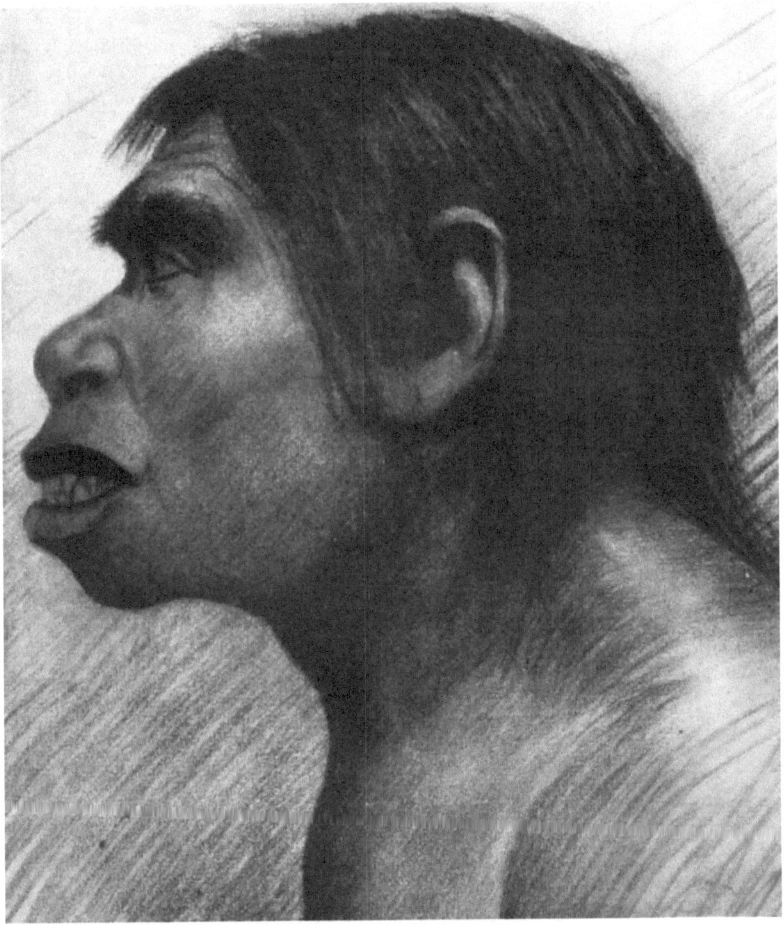

EARLIEST INHABITANT OF ENGLAND

(*See page* 263)

PLATE VII

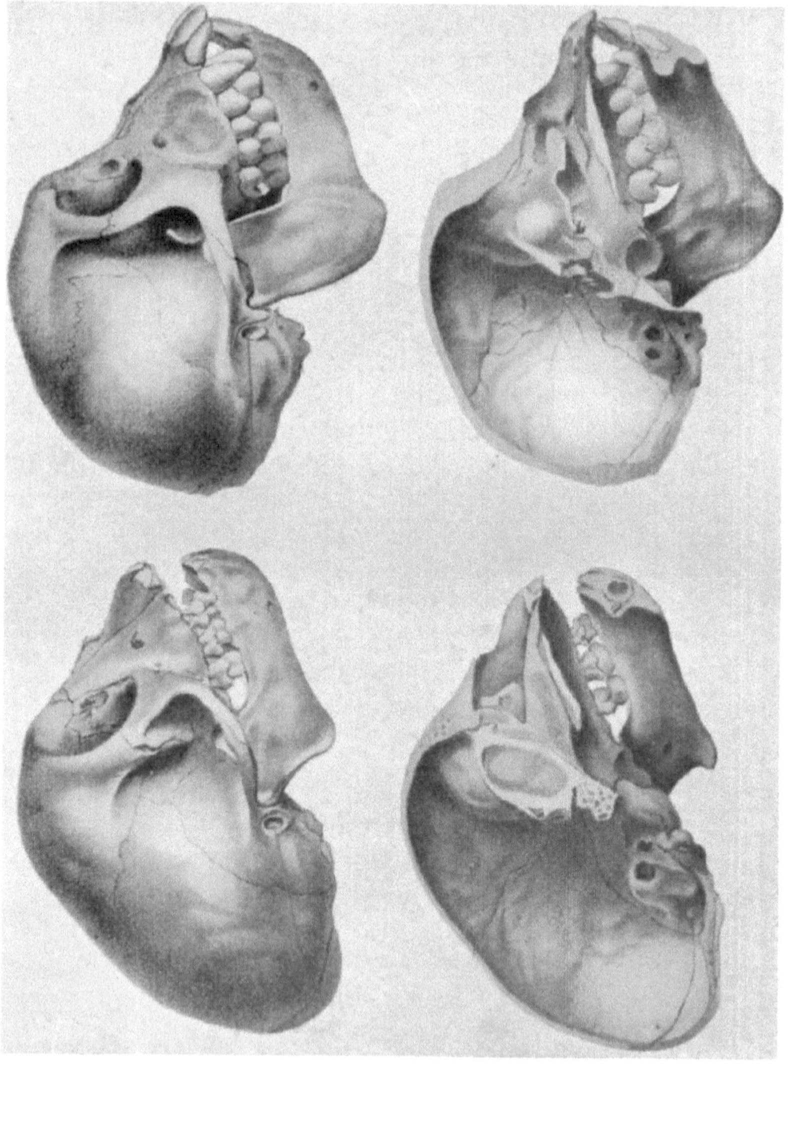

FEMALE AND MALE MONKEY SKULLS AND SECTION OF THEM

The female skull is longer posteriorly (*see page* 265)

by craniologists and anthropologists—will not furnish reliable data for the estimation of the intellectual superiority or inferiority of a race or individual.

Professor KARL PEARSON F.R.S., in a lecture at University College, London, 1902, stated that he had taken two standards of ability: (1) a youth's view of his own capacity, and (2) the teacher's view of his capacity. "In neither case", he said, was there "a sensible relation between ability and shape of the head *as judged by the cephalic index*." This is what we should expect. The cephalic index is a totally insufficient measure, and conveys, at best, mental power, without indicating what direction that power takes. It may be in ability; or, in the primary emotions and instincts. Professor Pearson concluded that there is no correlation of intellectual ability with the size of the entire head, a conclusion which is obvious; for the purely intellectual functions—as we shall prove in later chapters—are confined to the frontal region of the cortex, which, as I have said, constitutes about a third of the entire mass of the brain.

SIR CHARLES SHERRINGTON (*Lectures on Physiology for Teachers*, London, 1901) was, therefore, also quite correct in his observation that the brain may be wide or narrow, deep or flattened, the shape of the *entire* mass will not give any clue to the intellectual endowment of its former possessor.

A fact that is frequently overlooked by those craniologists who rely solely on the measurements of the circumference of the head, is that it has to be taken at a level of the skull which does not admit of growth; that is to say, slightly above the rigid base. On the other hand, the vault of the skull remains open, in two places at least, for some time after birth; and, *even in later life, it is still capable of an increased arching, to make room for increased brain-mass.*

Circumference alone, as a measure of the skull and its contents, is inadequate; not only because the brain has other, besides intellectual functions, but because it may grow in certain regions without affecting the circumferential measurement.

I have three female adult skulls in my collection; each one has the circumference of 524 millimetres, i.e. 20·6 inches, but the cubic capacity of

No. 1 is 1,390 cubic centimetres,
No. 2 is 1,550 cubic centimetres,
No. 3 is 1,420 cubic centimetres,

which shows a difference between skull No. 1 and skull No. 2 of 160 cubic centimetres, or 11·5 per cent.

We see, then, that the size of brain, unless it be abnormal, conveys no information; and it is not surprising that those anatomists, craniologists, and anthropologists who trusted to one measurement alone (of the circumference of the head), or relied on the cephalic index, have been unable to determine at what age the brain attains full development.

SÖMMERING supposed that the brain finished its growth as early as the third year. WENZEL, TIEDEMANN, HAMILTON, HAMMOND, DONALDSON, and LINCOLN thought the brain finished growing about the seventh year. IRELAND considered the period to be about ten or twelve years of age, and Sir WILLIAM TURNER considered development to cease about thirty years of age; while MEYNERT considered the brain to reach its greatest weight in the fortieth year. Others found that the brain goes on growing in size so long as we go on learning.

JOHN VENN and FRANCIS GALTON read a paper to the Anthropological Society, April 24, 1888, on *Head Growth* in Students at the University of Cambridge, containing the following conclusions:

1. Although it is pretty well ascertained that in the masses of the population the brain ceases to grow after the age of

nineteen, or even earlier, it is by no means so with University students.

2. That men who obtain high honours have, at the age of nineteen, considerably larger brains than others.

3. That at the age of twenty-five they have larger brains than others; but not to the same extent. In fact, their predominance is, by that time, diminished to one-half of what it was.

4. Consequently, "high honour" men are presumably, as a class, both precocious and more gifted, throughout, than others. We must, therefore, look upon eminent University success as a fortunate combination of these two helpful conditions.

As I have said, neither measuring nor weighing the entire brain, or estimating the skull capacity, can help us in judging intellectual ability, and the data supplied by anthropologists and craniologists can, therefore, convey little or nothing that is of value for the solution of this problem.

The following are the *skull capacities of some well-known men:*

	Cubic centimetres.
Age 39, Skobeleff, General	1,457
Age 43, Gambetta, Statesman	1,294
Age 51, Donizetti, Musician (died of G.P.I.)	1,391
Age 53, Thackeray, Author	1,644
Age 54, Descartes, Philosopher	1,700
Age 56, Broca, Anthropologist	1,485
Age 56, Dante, Poet	1,493
Age 57, Spurzheim, Phrenologist	1,559
Age 59, Dupuytren, Surgeon	1,436
Age 62, Bertillon, Anthropologist	1398,
Age 63, Cuvier, Naturalist	1,830
Age 64, Abercrombie, Physician	1,785
Age 66, Agassiz, Naturalist	1,512
Age 70, Liebig, Chemist	1,352
Age 70, Gall, Anatomist	1,692
Age 70, Petrarca, Poet	1,602
Age 74, La Fontaine, Author	1,950
Age 75, Grote, Historian	1,410

	Cubic centimetres.
Age 78, Gauss, Mathematician	1,492
Age 78, Tiedemann, Anatomist	1,254
Age 80, Scarpa, Surgeon	1,455
Age 82, Volta, Physicist	1,745

The following are the *brain weights of some well-known men:*

	Ounces.
Age 39. Skobeleff	51·5
Age 44, Gambetta	39
Age 46, Schiller	63
Age 53, Thackeray	58·5
Age 56, Spurzheim	55
Age 56. Dante	51·3
Age 58, Dupuytren	50·7
Age 59, Napoleon	57
Age 63, Cuvier	64·5
Age 64, Abercrombie	62·9
Age 67, Chalmers	53
Age 70, Daniel Webster	53·5
Age 70, Gall	42·25
Age 75, Grote	49·75
Age 78, Gauss	52·6
Age 80, Tiedemann	44·2
Age 80, Grant	45·5

Cromwell's brain was estimated at 78·8 oz.; but must be exaggerated, considering the size of the head as it appears in his portraits.

On the discovery of *Dante's* remains, at Ravenna, in 1865, the skull was pronounced to be ample, and exquisite in form. But its actual cubic capacity, and estimated brain weight, fall considerably below those of the heaviest brain weights of distinguished men.

Lord Byron died in Greece, in 1824, and English papers reported his brain weight as six medicinal pounds, a round figure, which renders it suspect of being inaccurate. In any case, it was either a Neapolitan or Venetian weight (the former 1,924

PLATE VIII

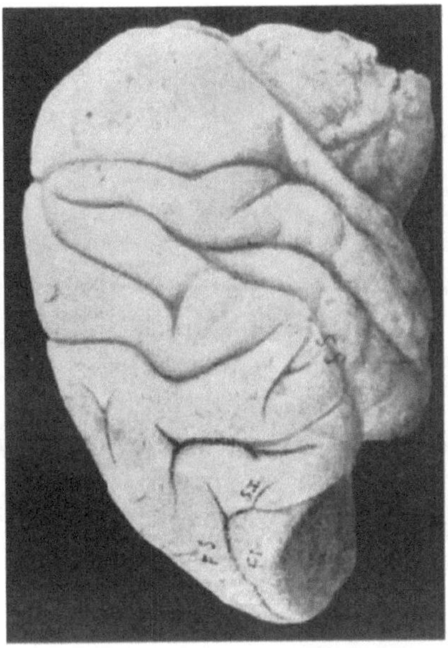

BRAIN OF A CEBUS, A LONG-TAILED MONKEY
Compare with human brain, Plate I

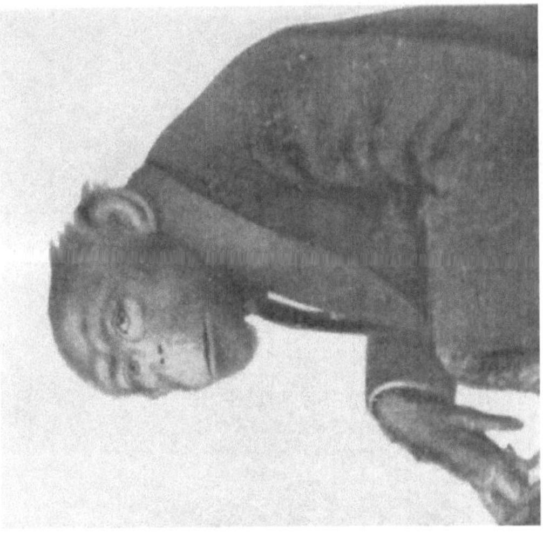

HEAD OF MONKEY
Notice small height of head

Plate IX

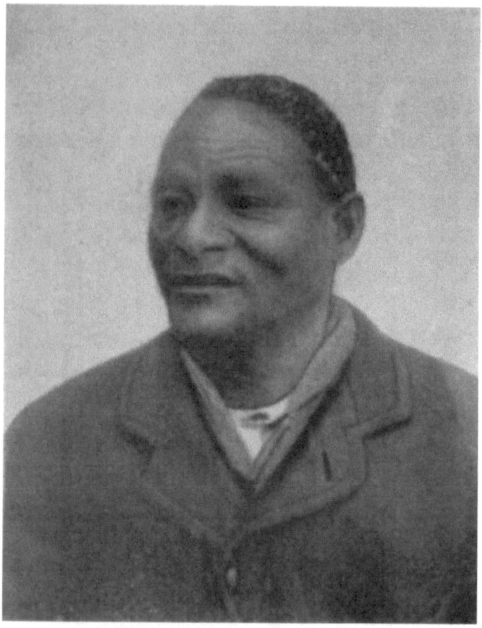

NATIVE CHIEF

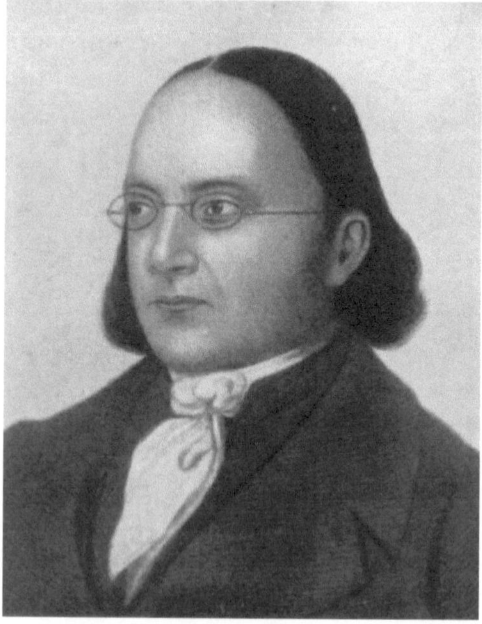

MISSIONARY

grammes, the latter 1,807 grammes); and it was stated that Byron's brain was in a hyperaemic condition, so that, probably, as I shall explain presently, no allowance was made for the blood which the brain contained.

Sir Walter Scott's portraits show an astoundingly large head. It is on record that the cranial arch, from ear to ear, as measured from the mastoid process, was 19 in.; whereas the average is only 14 in. The circumference of his head was 23·1 in., the longitudinal diameter 9 in., and the parietal 6·4 in. Yet, in the report of the post-mortem examination of Scott, the physicians stated "that the brain was not large". The peculiar shape of his skull was attributed to his lameness, dating from infancy, and due to water on the brain. SPITZKA, the American neurologist, made a similar statement about Cuvier, who had one of the heaviest brains on record, that it represented "not intellect, but healed-up hydrocephalus". Celebrities with large heads will not feel flattered by this explanation. Science is rarely complimentary, but this is well-nigh libellous?

If this explanation was correct, and the high head of Sir Walter Scott was due to hydrocephalus, how are we to account for the fact that all the other heads of creative geniuses, and men with lofty ideals and vivid imaginations, are also high, as may be seen from the illustrations?

The brain of Robert Burns measured, according to Sir ARTHUR KEITH, at least 1,680 cubic centimetres; 200 more than the average Scotsman. If the brain were merely an intellectual organ, it would be difficult to explain the extraordinary size of the brain of Robert Burns. One must infer that the brain is an emotional as well as an intellectual organ; and that such mass as that seen in the case of Burns is connected with the intensity of his emotions.

Few brain weights are taken nowadays, and the old results are almost worthless; for the number of weights taken was far too small, and greatly wanting in details. Moreover, the use of different standards of weights and measures, and of diverse material for determining the capacity of the skull in different countries, greatly complicates the researches of the craniologist. There was great variation, at one time, in the size of the inch alone. For example, the old French inches were about one-sixteenth longer than the English. Similarly, the pound weight varied in each country; so that little reliance can be placed on the published figures. In many cases the brain was not weighed at all, but only the internal capacity of the unearthed skull estimated, by filling it with millet or poppy seed, and then ascertaining the weight of the seed. Others employed shot, and others water. Even when the brain itself was weighed, we are left in doubt, as in the case of Byron, whether the brain was fresh, and still contained blood, or had the blood removed first. That is how we have obtained such vast differences as the abnormally heavy brain of the French naturalist, Cuvier, with $64\frac{1}{2}$ oz. and the abnormally light brain of Gambetta, the famous politician and orator, with 39 oz. The observations made of the weights of brains are unreliable, also, because they are frequently made only after the brains have lost from 27 per cent. to 40 per cent. in weight by their preservation in alcohol, and consequently have undergone some diminution in volume.

What we require is the weight of thousands of brains of healthy people—not insane and diseased—each brain being weighed as a whole, and each part—frontal, parietal, temporal, and occipital—separately, according to an agreed anatomical division. The frontal lobes may be highly developed, and the occipital lobes deficient. In another brain of exactly the same weight, the parietal lobes may be massive and the temporal lobes very small.

The most recent brain weight—that of Anatole France, the celebrated French author—was taken by Guillaume Louis and Dubreuil Chambardel, who read a paper on the subject at the Academy of Medicine in Paris on November 8, 1929. They reported that they found the weight of this brain to be 36 oz. (1,017 grammes) only, i.e. 13 oz. (343 grammes) less than that of the average citizen.

How unreliable—without the fullest details—these brain weights are, is shown by the careful weight taken of the brain of Helmholtz, who was distinguished for his wonderful researches in optics (*Zeitschrift für Psychiatrie*, 1899). The weight of his brain, including the blood coagulum, was 60 oz. (1,700 grammes). This being removed, the brain weighed 54 oz. (1,540 grammes); but so much blood remained, that it was estimated that 100 to 120 grammes (4 to 5 oz.) should be deducted. This would reduce the brain weight to the average, or slightly above it, namely, 49 to 50 oz. (1,420 to 1,440 grammes). Helmholtz had, therefore, a brain not much above the average weight.

Among the recent brain weights taken is an extraordinarily light one, that of *Ignaz von Dollinger*, a renowned Catholic theologian, which weighed 1,207 grammes; and another, also one of the *heaviest* on record, that of *Turgenieff*, the Russian novelist, which weighed 2,012 grammes.

The brain of Ernst Haeckel, the famous German naturalist, who died in 1912, in his eighty-sixth year, was examined by Professor F. Maurer of Jena. It weighed 1,575 grammes.

H. H. Donaldson (*Journal of Comparative Neurology*, 1928) weighed the brains of three eminent scholars: G. Stanley Hall, who died at the age of 78, had a brain weight of 1,412 grammes;

Professor William Osler, who died at the age of 70, 1,396 grammes; and Ed. Morse, who reached 87 years of age, had a brain 1,309 grammes in weight.

An average male brain weighs about 49 oz. and an average female brain 44 oz. PAPE and KOPELSKY give the weights as 1,363 grammes and 1,260 grammes respectively. The convoluted cortex weighs about 658 grammes (under 1½ lb.); but the nerve elements alone weigh only about 13 grammes (under ½ oz.). The human cortex is about 2 to 3 mm. thick (less than 1 in.), and contains, according to ECONOMO (see Chapter II), 14,000 million neurons; whereas the gorilla's cortex has been estimated to contain 3,000 to 4,000 millions of neurons only. There are 100 myelo-architectonic areas in the cortex of man; but only 32 corresponding areas can be distinguished in the lower monkeys, and 40 in the orang (according to MAUSS, *Journal of Psychology and Neurology*, 1908).

The orang and chimpanzee have cranial capacities of 26 and 27½ cubic in. respectively; while for normal man the lowest cranial capacity is 55 cubic in. The brain of the gorilla, which most closely resembles the human brain, weighs only 20 oz.; and those of the other anthropoid apes range from 12 to 16 oz. What is very important, in man's case, as compared with apes, apart from the increased dimensions and complexity, is the fact that man's brain goes on growing for a much longer time than that of the apes. In the first three months the human body, as a whole, adds 20 per cent. to its weight; the brain adds nearly 90 per cent. In less than 9 months, therefore, the weight of the brain is doubled; in 3 years it is trebled.

Sir ARTHUR KEITH points out ("*The Human Body*") that "*Man's brain is only about one-fifth of its adult weight at birth; that of the anthropoid is already two-thirds.* Man has to be

PLATE X

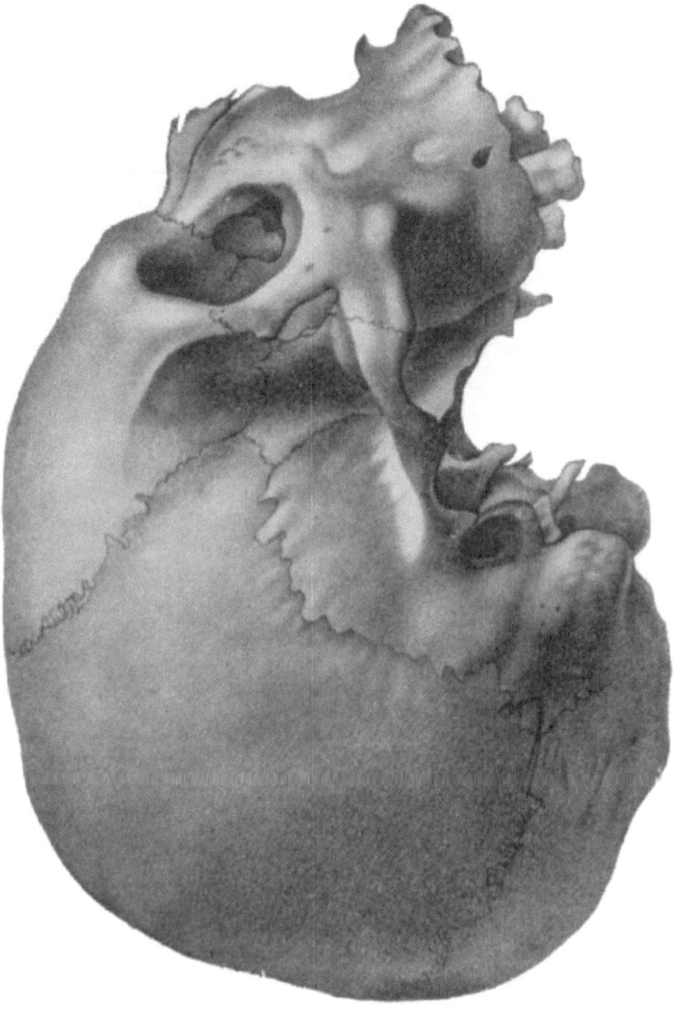

IDIOT SKULL
Compare with ordinary skull, Plate IV

PLATE XI

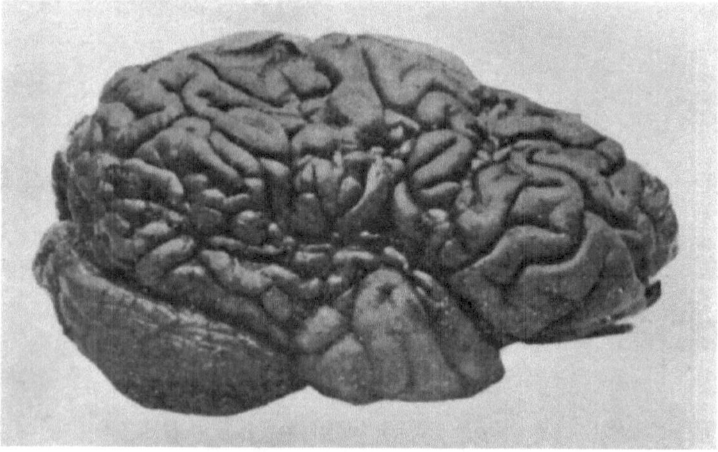

IDIOT BRAIN

(*See page* 93)

The reader should compare this brain with a normal one, and the skull and head of an idiot with those of an average man or of a man of genius, as shown in this book; for according to the following quotation, taken from a textbook by a distinguished psychological writer and University Lecturer, our students are still taught:—

"Between the brain of Einstein and that of an idiot there is no perceptible difference; at least it is not a difference of such a kind as to enable the physiologist to tell which brain is Einstein's and which is the idiot's."(!)

sheltered and educated; the anthropoid baby has to face the realities of life soon after birth. By the end of the second year the human brain has reached two-thirds of its adult size; it has then reached the same relative degree of development that the anthropoid has reached at birth." We see, then, that the human child, with prolonged infancy and prolonged play-period, would retain longer than in most cases what we might call "an open mind". In other words, it remains, for an unusually long time, very "educable"; with ample opportunities for testing idiosyncrasies.

The following figures of HERMANN WELCKER exhibit the cranial capacity in man at different ages, and, consequently, the progressive volume of his brain:

	MALE. Cubic centimetres.	FEMALE. Cubic centimetres.
New-born infant	400	360
At two months	540	510
At one year	900	850
At three years	1,080	1,010
At ten years	1,360	1,250
From twenty to sixty years	1,450	1,300

WEISBACH obtained the following weights of the brains of males between the ages of ten and ninety years, showing the increase in the *weight of the brain* up to middle age and the decline of its mass in senility.

	Grammes.
10–19 years of age	1,270
20–29 years of age	1,355
30–59 years of age	1,375
60–90 years of age	1,349

Comparisons are frequently made between European and savage brains; but such comparisons, to be of value, should be made between savage brains and those of unskilled workmen, or vagrants; for the educated man has the advantage of the accumulated knowledge and benefits of civilisation in general. Still, there may be races with inherited brains of greater capacity than their needs, in less civilised circumstances, may require. An exact equivalent to this may be seen in the feeble intellectuality of many of the peasants and lower classes among the civilised nations of modern times. The capacity is there, but latent. Hence it happens, not infrequently, that a youth born of such parents becomes, if educated, a distinguished citizen.

Similar remarks are applicable to the skulls of prehistoric races, as it would appear that evolution had done the major part of its work in brain development long before the days of neolithic civilisation. Some of the skulls of fossil men are of large size, but chiefly in the posterior region. It would seem that the growth of the frontal region of the brain has tended to diminish the posterior development. Until localisation of brain functions makes greater progress, it is futile to speculate to any great extent on the relative sizes of skulls of different races, either in present or prehistoric times.

Plate XII

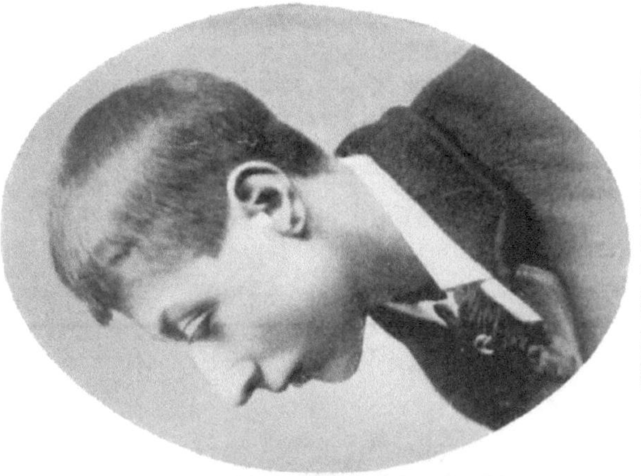

HEAD OF A BACKWARD BOY

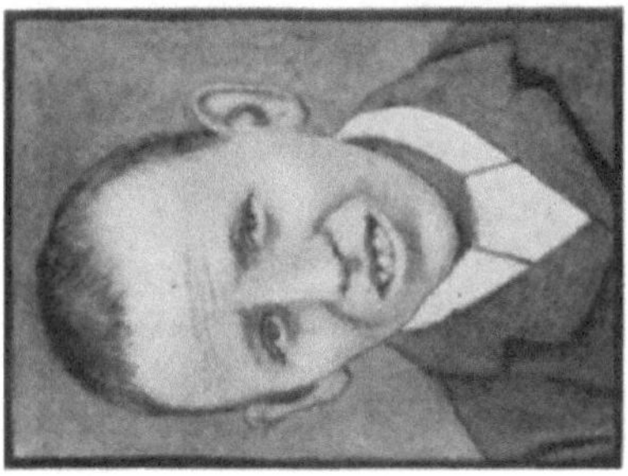

HEAD OF AN IMBECILE

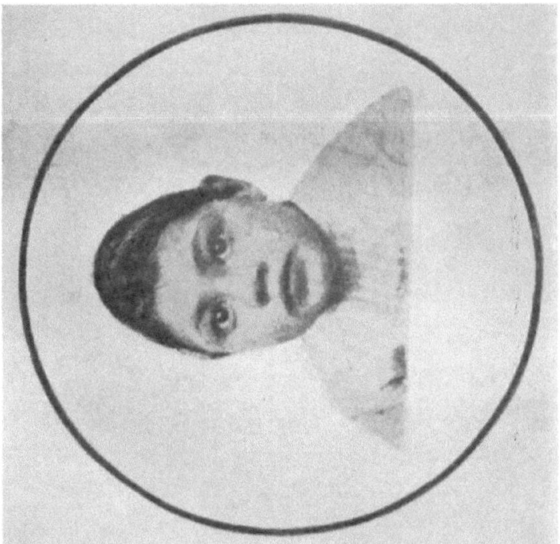

HEAD OF A MICROCEPHALOUS IDIOT

CHAPTER VI

SENSORY DISTURBANCES, DEPRESSION, AND ANXIETY IN LESIONS OF THE PARIETAL LOBES

It has been shown, in the preceding chapters, that research into the functions of the brain has failed, so far, to reveal their connection with mental activities; and that, chiefly, because mind and intellect were considered identical. In point of fact, however, all mental manifestation has its origin in the emotions and instincts, which, so far, have been practically neglected, or, at least, not considered to be functions of the cortex of the brain. Now, the brain is, primarily, an organ for the preservation of life; and to this end a number of instincts are needed.

If we take the most primitive living being, an amoeba—which consists of nothing more than a mere bit of protoplasm—and touch some part of it, it will withdraw that part instantaneously; thus protecting itself from possible injury. Higher up in the scale of animal life, when a nervous system, and, finally, a brain has developed, we find a special region, corresponding to the parietal lobes in the human brain, set apart, which appears to react whenever the animal experiences a disagreeable sensation, or perceives or suspects danger, and, simultaneously, an emotion is aroused, an unpleasant, depressing emotion—an emotion of anxiety, fear, or terror—according to the degree of pain or danger whether threatened or imagined. In man, if the anxiety persists, we may get a mental condition known as "melancholia".

The parietal lobes are generally regarded as containing the centres of sensation; and disturbances of sensation are common in melancholia and in all lesions of the lateral aspect of the parietal lobes.

J. A. Lockhart Clarke has said "that the anterior and posterior lobes have different functions is certain, as the convolutions of the cerebral regions have different structure".

Bernhard Gudden declared the anterior half of the brain to be concerned with motion, and the posterior half with sensation.

Luigi Luciani and Giuseppe Seppilli were of opinion that the fusion of sensory centres takes place in the parietal lobes.

Chas. K. Mills (*Philadelphia Medical Journal*, 1901) held that cerebral tumours in the parietal region render patients abnormally emotional.

Francesco Durante declared the posterior lobes to be the centre for general sensibility, and believed them to be involved in melancholia.

R. v. Krafft-Ebing considered melancholia a form of neurosis, or psychical neuralgia, of the sensory centres of the brain. Undoubtedly, melancholia gives rise to a psychical hyperaesthesia.

From time immemorial intellectual functions have been associated with the brain; but not so the feelings. Yet, whether we assume that they arise through external stimuli, through bodily sensations, or through ideas of our own, communicated to us, each rudimentary feeling—if there is anything like order in the nervous system—must have a centre in some group of nerve cells, from which it can set the rest of the brain into activity, and produce its bodily manifestation. Though the effect of such an impulse may be an all-pervading one, there must be a centre from which the impulse starts. This has been recognised from time to time by individual observers, who located a general region for feelings in the optic thalamus at the base of the brain.

Henry Head and Gordon Holmes regard the optic

thalamus as the central basis of emotive reaction; but all they have actually proved is that the optic thalamus is the central organ for the conveying of sensations—for painful and tactile impulses, the appreciation of heat and cold, the vibration sense, sense of position and movement, and for sensations of pleasure and discomfort in general.

It has since been demonstrated that projection fibres go from the optic thalamus to the cortex of the parietal lobes (and to a lesser extent to other parts); and it will be shown by hundreds of cases of lesions within that area, that they give rise to the emotion of fear. The emotion may be caused by sensations in the thalamus, or it may arise mentally, from the perception of danger; and the subsequent reaction may be conducted to the optic thalamus by the bundle of fibres connecting that part of the cortex with the nucleus ruber and Monakow's rubro-spinal bundle (as demonstrated by Déjerine).

William Elder (*Studies in Psychology*, 1927) pointed out that the thalamus has direct connections with various parts of the cortex, both through afferent nerves to the cortex and efferent nerves from the cortex; and that there must, therefore, be very intimate associations of the thalamus and cortex: the thalamus transmitting nerve impulses to the cortex, and the cortex transmitting nerve impulses to the thalamus.

The emotions, primarily, are cerebral, i.e. mental states; the visceral expressions being purely secondary. Let anyone study the cases of fear after head injury, and he must become convinced that this theory is right, and that James, Lange, and Sergi, who held that the emotions were secondary to the actions of the viscera, must be wrong. The decorticated dog and the decerebrated cat still have the power to express fear, but they lack the parts of the mechanism that elicit response upon the application of fear-producing stimuli.

SIR CHARLES SHERRINGTON (*The Integrative Action of the Nervous System*, 1906) has shown that, if an experiment be performed on an animal, in such a manner as to remove all sensation of the bodily organs, skin, and muscles—upon which James laid so much stress in his peripheral theory of the emotions—the animal, thus experimented upon, shows all grades of emotional expression. Here, the brain was left intact, but the peripheral sensations were obliterated; yet, no alteration occurred in the emotional character of the animal. As CORIAT says (*Abnormal Psychology*, Boston, 1910): "To the ordinary individual, this central theory of the emotions is the most logical one; he trembles because he is afraid, he strides because he is angry, etc."

That the parietal lobes are, in some way, associated with the emotion of fear is supported by experimental evidence.

HERMANN MUNK (*Über die Funktionen der Grosshirnrinde*, Berlin, 1881) found that, if the *gyrus angularis* is removed from both hemispheres of the brain in dogs, "when the animal had recovered from the inflammatory reaction, the sight of the whip, which had formerly frightened the animal away to a corner, had now not the least terrifying effect". A monkey, similarly operated upon, suffered, consequently, from "non-perception of obstacles and dangers".

FERRIER observed that: "The animal whose left angular gyrus was destroyed moved only unwillingly; and when it was obliged to, *it ran its head full tilt against everything that came in its way*. When both angular gyri were destroyed, the animal *paid no attention to threats* and grimaces."

THOS. HUXLEY, in an address to the British Association for the Advancement of Science, in 1874, quoted the remarkable case of a man observed by him, who had been shot in the left parietal bone. This man had fits of trance, when, "if you put an obstacle in his way, he knocks against it, feels it, and goes to one side".

F. L. Goltz and Beatson found that destruction of the posterior lobes, in dogs and sheep, causes these animals *no longer to be frightened by objects* that had produced terror, previous to the operation. Dogs, which were lively and active before the operation, became quiet and apathetic, and their intellect was inhibited.

Jac. Moleschott noticed that, immediately after destroying, in pigeons, that portion of the brain corresponding to the parietal lobes in man, they showed a *total imperception of danger.*

Albert E. Eulenburg found by experiments on dogs that stimulation of the parietal region produced irritation of the vaso-motor nerves, together with such symptoms as sudden emptying of the bowels, which we frequently observe in fear.

In lesions of the parietal lobes, there is an unreasonable apprehensive depression, which retards thoughts and movements, and interferes greatly with self-control, without impairing the reasoning power. Whereas joyful emotions accelerate the course of ideas, anxiety, fear, grief, and all depressing emotions, inhibit intellectual processes.

The intellect remains intact, but gets restricted to the patient's own woes, and as every exertion augments the distress, such patients avoid all occupation, become inert and indecisive, and brood over their own sadness. Fear and apprehension shade and modify the reminiscences of the past, exaggerate dangers, and distort reality. Thus, a just and rational view of life is no longer taken. The subject is generally acutely conscientious, and full of self-depreciation; he distresses himself, needlessly, with worries, the unreasonableness of which is appreciated by him, but cannot be got rid of. Other feelings are paralysed; consequently, the patient becomes indifferent towards those persons and things which he used to hold in affection. The feeling of fear is so accentuated, that any trifling mistake made is exaggerated, and self-accusations follow, which, however, are not delusions, but simply reasons to account for the depressed feeling and state of anxiety. As the disease progresses, the patient anticipates dreadful consequences of his past errors; he is therefore unhappy, sleeps badly, weeps, sobs, sighs, groans, laments his cruel fate, and wishes to be dead. Suicide is common.

The parietal lobes, as I have shown, are connected with the involuntary (sympathetic) nervous system, which will explain why lesions of the parietal lobes so often give rise to anxious mental states, depression, and peculiar sensations from the bodily organs, not infrequently resulting in delusions about them (so common in melancholia). The cerebro-spinal system is rendered inactive; hence the muscular languor, lassitude, and loss of all sense of energy.

On the other hand, the frontal lobes (as has been shown in Chapter II) contain the centres for the voluntary (cerebro-spinal) nervous system, and this will explain (as will be proved in succeeding chapters) why lesions of the frontal lobes usually give rise to great physical and mental activity, and to cheerful mental states, the sympathetic system making no impression on the cortex for the time being, and, thus, no impression on consciousness.

Fear acts on the sympathetic nervous system, and renders the cerebro-spinal nerves inactive; hence, the muscular languor, lassitude, and loss of all sense of energy.

Frequently, there is a condition resembling what is called "apraxia", namely, an inability to execute the movement required to carry out a definite action; although there is no paralysis. This muscular inability is acknowledged to take place in lesions of the parietal lobes. In this malady an erect figure is never seen. The subject may remain fixed in one attitude, in an acute state of fear. In another degree of melancholia he may be restless; but this restlessness is brought about by the involuntary nervous system, and is quite different from the maniacal restlessness which originates in the voluntary or cerebro-spinal nervous system.

Pure melancholia being an emotional, and not an intellectual disease, it is not surprising to discover that JULIUS JENSEN (*Archiv. für Psychiatrie*, Vol. XX), who examined 453 brains of insane patients, found that *in melancholia the frontal lobes are not involved*, and that W. T. TIGGES (*Allg. Zeitschrift für Psychiatrie*, 1888) made the same observation. The latter said: "In melancholia, there is no wasting of the frontal lobes—they retain their weight; in mania, there is some loss of weight; in general paralysis, the loss is the greatest."

Another indirect proof of the correctness of this localisation has been furnished by C. BESTA (*Riv. di Pat. nerv. e. ment.*, 1922), who found that "the intellect is not impaired, even with severe lesions of the parietal lobes, so long as they are limited to this region".

This view was also expressed, long ago, by SCHRÖDER VAN DER KOLK, in his textbook on *Mental Disorders* (1852), in which he said: "In insanity proper, in cases of confusion of ideas, and of insanity of exaltation, I have always found the anterior lobes of the brain suffering; but, on the contrary, in the melancholic, and in those who condemned themselves, with or without religious delusions, I have found the upper and posterior parts of the hemispheres diseased; and that, in the latter cases, the understanding often showed no trace of disturbance, inasmuch as the individuals judged correctly, and disputed acutely. In those who, at last, perished with dementia, I never found the anterior parts of the lobes intact; they were always adherent to the pia mater, and this could not be removed without injuring the grey cortex."

There is ample material to prove the relation of melancholic states of mind to pathological conditions of the parietal lobes —more particularly, of the *angular and supra-marginal convolutions*; but it may extend right down to the occipital lobes.

Allowance must be made for tumours of the brain, which in the advanced stage often cause considerable intra-cranial tension, and thus give rise to symptoms of neighbouring areas. This will account for tumours of the temporal lobes giving rise, though rarely, to symptoms of melancholia. On the other hand, melancholia does occur, not infrequently, in cases of frontal lesions; but only in people already hyperconscientious, hypersensitive, and fearful. The frontal lobes, as will be explained, act normally as an inhibitory organ; and when this inhibition is lost, the natural dispositions become more acute. At the same time, such symptoms as apathy and lethargy, in advanced lesions of the frontal lobes, must not be mistaken for signs of melancholia.

Sometimes the whole brain may appear to be affected. There may be a general anaemia of the brain, causing a so-called inanition melancholia. Toxins, also, may cause melancholia. But, in all these conditions, it will be found that the disposition to this mental trouble was already existent, and became manifest only owing to these physical causes.

A fact worth noting is that *visual hallucinations are common to lesions of the parietal and occipital lobes*, and in melancholia; whilst *auditory hallucinations most frequently occur in lesions of the temporal lobes*, and acute mania.

Alienists have doubted whether melancholia, as an independent disease, ever exists. In my own experience, it does. But even if it did not, states of depression, with anxious emotion, might still take their origin in the parietal lobe; as the evidence which I am about to submit indicates.

Examples of Lesions of the Parietal Lobes followed by Abnormal Fear, Anxiety, and Melancholia

I. *Surgical Treatment of Parietal Injuries Resulting in Recovery*

By the Author.	Lancet, 1907. Six years after injury.
G. H. Hume.	Ibidem, 1908.
Wm. MacEwen.	Ibidem, 1888, *Two cases.*
Geo. E. Wherry.	British Medical Journal, 1863.
H. Handford.	Ibidem, 1899.

G. Mackenzie Bacon.	Journal of Mental Science, 1881. One year after injury.
W. B. Fletcher.	American Journal of Insanity, 1886–7. *Five cases.* One, six years; another, eight years after injury.
L. V. Briggs.	Philadelphia Medical News, Vol. XIV. Five years after injury.
J. E. Chambers.	Report of Cosmop. Sanat., St. Louis, 1906.
H. A. Powell.	Surgical Aspect of Traumatic Insanity, 1893. Seven years after injury.
Geo. W. Gale.	New York Medical Journal, 1895. Four years after injury.
Chas. Phelps.	Traumatic Injuries to the Brain, 1898.
Wm. Sharpe.	Diag. and Treatment of Brain Injuries, 1920.
Rathmann.	Vierteljahrschrift f. gerichtl. Medizin, 1901.
P. Stetter.	Centralblatt f. Chirurgie, 1892. Eleven years after injury.
J. M. Köppe.	Deutsch. Arch. f. Klin. Medizin, Vol. XIII. *Two cases.* One, four years after injury.
Hahn.	Allg. Zeitschr. f. Psychiatrie, 1892.
Boubila & Pantaloni.	Gazette des Hôpitaux, 1892.
Philippe Rey.	Report of Alienist Congress, Lyons, 1891.
H. Duret.	Traumatismes Cranio-Cérébraux, 1919.
Daniel Mollière.	Report of the French Surg. Congr. 1885. *Two cases.*
Fenoglio.	Archiv. di Psichiatria, 1884.
Fenoglio.	Bologna Rivista Clinica, 1887.
T. Riboli.	Phil. Seb. Vol. I. Four years after injury.
M. Gamberini.	Bull. d. Science mediche di Torino, Vol. I.
W. Sharpe.	Diagnosis and Treatment of Brain Injuries, 1920. *Three cases.*
Rudolf Ahlers.	Über Schädelschüsse, Berlin, 1916. *Four cases.* Nr. 51, 65, 88, and 105; and *five cases* through shot in occiput; also, *one* from a sabre cut: "mentally depressed, given to plaintive crying".

II. *Examples of Parietal Injuries with Melancholia not Surgically Treated*

Ernest Tredinnick.	British Medical Journal, 1900.
G. Alder Blumer.	American Journal of Insanity, 1892.
S. V. Clevenger.	Alienist and Neurologist, 1888.
W. Wagner.	Volkmann's Klinische Vorträge, 1886. *Two cases.*
W. Wagner.	Vierteljahrschr. f. gerichtl. Medizin, 1888.
L. v. Muralt.	Allg. Zeitschrift f. Psychiatrie, 1900.
R. Thomsen.	Charité Annalen, Vol. XIII.
R. Thomsen.	Archiv. f. Psychiatrie, 1884. *Two cases.*
L. Löwenfeld.	Ibidem, 1898.
Ludwig Bruns.	Neurologisches Centralblatt, 1889.
G. Huguenin.	Krankheiten des Nervensystems, 1880.
Hermann Demme.	Militär-Chirurgische Studien, 1864.
Paul Schüller.	Psychosen nach Kopfverletzungen, 1882. *Two cases.*
Ludwig Schlager.	Zeitschr. d. Ges. d. Aerzte z. Wien, 1857. *Two cases.*
Eugène Azam.	Archives Gén. de Médecine, 1881.
Deroubaix.	Belgique Médicale, 1906.
C. T. Dent.	Polyclinic. "After-effects of Head Injuries." *Several cases.*
Erich Feuchtwanger.	"Funktionen des Stirnhirns", 1922. *Two cases* of melancholia due to injury extending to parietal lobes. Nos. 14 and 19.

III. *Examples of Melancholia with so-called "Psychical" Blindness*

Chas. W. Burr.	Journ. of Nerv. and Mental Dis., 1897.
Kuczinski.	Neurologisches Centralblatt, 1910.
G. Anton.	Wiener Klinische Wochenschrift, 1889.
C. S. Freud.	Archiv. f. Psychiatrie, 1889. *Two cases.*
J. M. Charcot.	Progress Médical, 1883.
Cotard.	Archives de Neurologie, 1884.
A. Chauffard.	Revue de Médecine, 1881.

IV. *Examples of Melancholia due to Parietal Injuries, with Post-mortem Evidence*

T. Crisp English.	Lancet, 1904. *Three cases.*
John Gay.	Ibidem, 1879. *Committed suicide.*
T. S. Clouston.	Journal of Mental Science, 1872. *Two cases.*
W. J. Mickle.	Ibidem, 1883.
C. W. Burr.	Journal of Nerv. and Mental Disease, 1898.
John P. Gray.	American Journal of Insanity, 1876.
M. Dinkler.	Deutsche Zeitschr. f. Nervenheilkunde, 1895.
J. v. Maschka.	Ger.-mediz. Urteile, 1873.
J. v. Maschka.	Prager medizinische Wochenschrift, 1897.
Landerer & Lutz.	Christophsbad Asylum Report, 1878.
E. Sommer.	Casuistik d. Gehirnverletzungen, 1874.
Stolper.	Vierteljahrschr. f. ger. Medizin, 1897.
E. Mendel.	Progressive Paralyse, 1880.
C. J. Ellefsen.	Norsk. Magaz. f. Laegevdensk, 1896.
L. Marchand.	Nouvelle Iconographie de la Salpétrière, 1910.

V. *Examples of Melancholia due to Softening of the Parietal Lobes.*

D. Ferrier.	West Riding Lunatic Asylum Medical Reports, 1874.
P. Nicol.	Ibidem, 1872.
Percy Smith.	Journal of Mental Science, 1890.
James Shaw.	Brain, 1882.
James Shaw.	Ibidem, 1895.
J. Lockhart Clarke.	British Medical Journal, 1874.
W. T. Gairdner.	Ibidem, 1875.
W. Grant Cooper.	State Hospitals Bulletin, 1897.
E. Kundt.	Allg. Zeitschr. f. Psychiatrie, 1894. *Several cases.*
A. Rosenthal.	Centralblatt f. Nervenheilkunde, 1889.
Voisin & Burlureaux.	De la Mélancolie, 1880. *Numerous cases.*
J. Luys.	L'Encéphale, 1881. *Two cases.*
F. Lallemand.	Rech. anat.-path. s. l'Encéphale, Vol. II.

VI. *Examples of Tumours of the Parietal Lobes Causing Melancholia*

Sir William Broadbent	Lancet, 1874.
Jas. Crichton Browne	British Medical Journal, 1873.
T. R. Glynn.	Ibidem, 1878.
Anderson.	Ibidem, 1889.
P. Nicol.	West Riding Lunatic Asy. Med. Reports, 1872.
T. S. Clouston.	Journal of Mental Science, 1879.
Wm. Boyd.	Ibidem, 1873.
L. Pierce Clark.	Journal of Nerv. and Mental Dis., 1895.
M. Bernhardt.	Allg. Zeitschr. f. Psychiatrie, 1886.
Th. Sarlan.	Ibidem, 1886.
C. v. Monakow.	Archiv. f. Psychiatrie, 1881.
T. Zacher.	Ibidem, 1888.
H. Oppenheim.	Ibidem, 1890.
B. Pfeifer.	Ibidem, 1910.
E. Mendel.	Neurologisches Centralblatt, 1882.
Stein.	Ibidem, 1897.
G. Anton.	Ibidem, 1900.
Touche.	Ibidem, 1900. *Crying Fits.*
H. Oppenheim.	Charité Annalen, Vol. X.
Ludwig Bruns.	Jahresber. f. Neur. u. Psychiatrie, 1898.
Tambroni.	Ibidem, 1898.
R. Virchow.	Onkologie, Vol. II.
H. Baruk.	"Les Troubles Mentaux dans les Tumeurs Cérébrales," 1926, Case 24. "Patient sad; very depressed; wanted to be alone."
Petrina.	Prager Vierteljahrschrift, 1874.
L. Manouvrier.	Bull. de la Soc. d'Anthrop. de Paris, 1885.
H. D. Dagonet and P. Rey.	Annales Médico-Psychologiques, 1882.
Marot.	Bull. de la Soc. Anatom., 1875.
Lwoff.	Lésions Circonscrites, 1890. *Crying Fits.*
Gianelli.	Policlinico, 1897. *Two cases.*

VII. *Examples of Tumours of the Occipital Lobes Causing Melancholia*

Berthold Pfeifer.	Allg. Zeitschrift f. Psychiatrie, 1910.
Jany.	Centralblatt f. Augenheilkunde, 1882. *Excess of grief, weeping.*
H. Schule.	Sectionsergebnisse bei Geisteskrankheiten, 1874. *Insane grief at loss of child.*
Paul Schuster.	Hirntumoren, 1902. *Anxious, melancholic, and crying constantly.*

VIII. *Examples of Cases of Melancholia due to Haemorrhage into Parietal Region (Haematoma of Dura Mater)*

Gairdner, Robertson and Coats.	British Medical Journal, 1875.
G. H. Hume.	Lancet, 1908.
W. J. Mickle.	Journal of Mental Science, 1880.
J. Wiglesworth.	Ibidem, 1888.
H. D. MacPhail.	Ibidem, 1915.
D. J. Cunningham.	Journal of Anatomy and Physiology, 1879.
Pliny Earle.	American Journal of Insanity, Vol. II.
S. G. Webber.	Boston Medical and Surgical Journal, 1883.
F. C. Hoyt.	Medical Record, 1892.
Rudolf Arndt.	Archiv. f. path. Anatomie, 1871.
C. Fröhlich.	Allg. Zeitschr. f. Psychiatrie, 1875.
Brie.	Neurologisches Centralblatt, 1897.
F. A. Amelung.	Bericht uber das Hofheimer Spital.
Joffé	Vierteljahrsschrift f. Psychiatrie, 1867.
Seidlitz.	Zeitschrift f.d. ger. Medizin.
L. Meyer.	Archiv. f. Psychiatrie, 1872.
H. Aubanel.	Annales Médico-Psychologiques, Vol. II. *Several cases.*
J. B. Bouillaud.	Ibidem. *Several cases.*
J. L. B. Cruveilhier.	Ibidem. *Several cases.*
P. Rey.	Ibidem, Vol. VIII.
L. F. Calmeil.	Traité d. Malad. Infl. d. Cerveau. *Several cases.*

Aug. Voisin and Burlureaux.	De la Mélancolie, 1880. *Numerous cases.*
S. Pozzi.	L'Encéphale, 1883.

IX. *Examples of Cases of Melancholia Followed by Symmetrical Atrophy of the Parietal Bones* (see Illustration)

R. Virchow.	Verhandlungen der Phys. Med. Gesellschaft zu Würzburg, 1854.
Rudolf Bloch.	Prager Medizinische Wochenschrift, 1897. *Two cases.*
Ludwig Meyer.	Archiv. f. Psychiatrie, 1872.
Rossbach.	Deutsches Archiv. f. Klinische Medizin, 1890.
H. Schüle.	Sektionsergebnisse bei Geisteskranken, 1874.
W. B. Pritchard.	Journal of Nervous and Mental Disease, 1890.
H. Voppel.	Allg. Zeitschrift f. Psychiatrie, Vol. XIV.
W. Fränkel.	Ibidem, 1887.
F. A. Kirchhoff.	Ibidem, 1883.

X. *Examples of Cases of Melancholia with Abnormal Development of the Parietal Lobes*

J. E. D. Esquirol.	Maladies Mentales. *Several cases.*
M. Rivet.	Bull. de la Société Anat. de Paris, 1887.
A. Campbell Clark.	Journal of Mental Science, 1879.
H. Voppel.	Allg. Zeitschrift f. Psychiatrie, Vol. XIV. *Four cases.*

Extraordinary dimensions across the parietal bones in chronic melancholics, judging by my own observations, are not uncommon; but, hitherto, have not been considered worth consideration, even when noticed.

Sufficient evidence has been given, I hope, to prove that the supra-marginal and angular convolutions, and the parieto-occipital area, are, in some way, connected with the emotion of fear and with the production of anxious states of mind.

Plate XIII

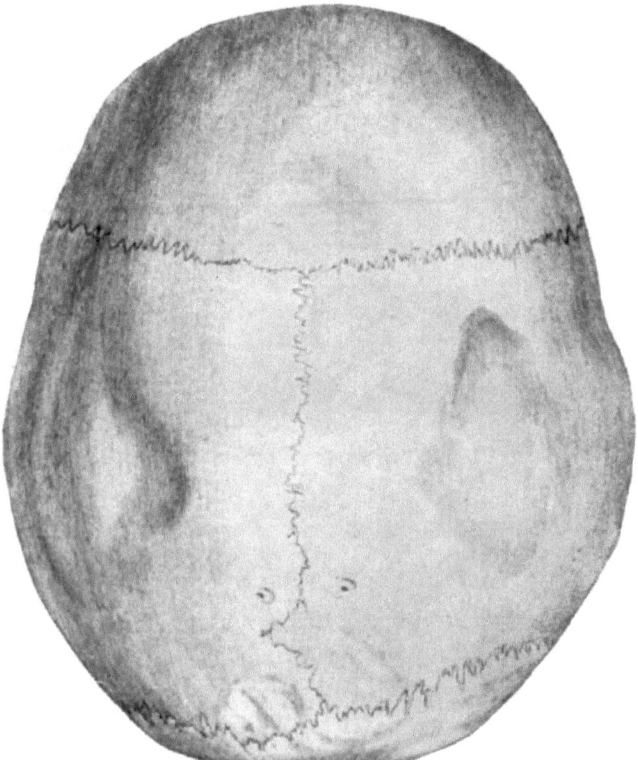

SYMMETRICAL WASTING OF SKULL

(*See page* 120)

Plate XIV

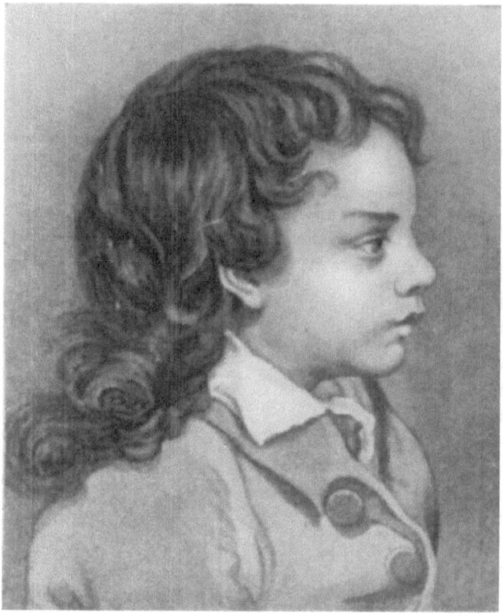

CHATTERTON, THE POET

Committed suicide at eighteen

The head is large in the frontal and parietal areas (*see page* 121)

I have quoted about thirty cases of parietal tumours with symptoms of melancholia. Paul Schuster (*Psychische Störungen bei Hirntumoren*, 1902), who had examined the symptoms accompanying parietal tumours (which I first announced in a small pamphlet of mine, published by me in 1898) stated that "neither progressive paralysis, nor paranoia, nor mania, ever occur in such cases; but that *they are mostly accompanied by states of depression*". He saw nothing improbable in my localisation of melancholia in this region.

Chas. K. Mills (*Philadelphia Medical Journal*, 1901) also declared that *tumours of the parietal lobes are accompanied by emotional depression.*

Anglade (*L'Encéphale*, 1921) confirmed, too, the observation that melancholia is often a symptom of parietal lesions.

Every case of melancholia is a potential suicide, and in the detailed history of the cases quoted, which I have given in my earlier books, it may be seen that a large number of these patients had attempted self-destruction, no matter whether the lesion was one due to injury, tumour, or other causes. W. C. Sullivan (*Lancet*, 1911), however, stated that "Actual suicide appears to be a very rare occurrence in cerebral tumour; I have found only one case mentioned in the literature of the disease (a case reported by Rey, quoted by Bernhardt, *Beiträge zur Symptomatologie und Diagnostik der Gehirngeschwülste*, Berlin, 1881); and in a series of 1,700 post-mortem examinations of suicides reported by Pilcs (*Ann. Méd.-Psych.*, 1908), new growths were found in the brain in only three cases."

Aug. Voisin read a paper on "The Suicidal Tendency" to the Academy of Medicine in Paris, in 1882, in which he declared that his observations led him to the conclusion that the particular part of the brain which gave *the tendency and impulse to suicide, so common in melancholia, is in the parietal lobes.*

Dr. Richard Eager (*Journal of Mental Science*, 1920), in his report on Head Injuries received by soldiers in the recent war, stated that he had had only three cases of parietal injury in his own care.

The *first* case mentioned was that of a man who had been wounded by a shell splinter "just above the pinna of the right ear", and, therefore, not in the parietal, but in the temporal region; and the mental change exhibited corresponded to that described in lesions of that area (see next chapter).

The *second* case was that of a boy, age nineteen, wounded by a bullet over the upper part of the parietal region which, in my opinion, corresponds to the posterior end of the frontal lobes, and so did the symptoms exhibited, as described in Chapter XI. The boy had had a record of good conduct all his life, and now became "a notorious liar, and full of deceit in every way".

The *third* case was that of a man below average intelligence, and should not have been included.

One case was returned as "psychasthenia", but seems to have been really one of "morbid fears". This patient suffered from "syphilophobia", which developed some months after a bullet wound in the posterior part of the left parietal region.

The most interesting thing, however, is that Dr. Eager found among his cases only two patients with occipital lesions of a serious character and both of them were "mentally melancholics", and had attempted suicide. This is a confirmation of the theory I have explained in this chapter, and is important in view of the fact of Dr. Eager stating that he could find no evidence for my localisations.

"The two cases whose injuries (of the occipital region)

were of a most serious character were both right-sided injuries, and both, mentally, *melancholics*. One was subsequently admitted to hospital, in a state of acute melancholia, having made an attempt to end his misery by strangulation with his puttees. The other case was one in which there was extensive loss of bony protection at the back of the skull. This man, during examination, admitted that he had contemplated suicide."

Were the evidence I have produced in this chapter better known and applied, it would not be necessary to have recourse to such a spectacle as the following occurrence presents. The report, which I give verbatim, refers to two patients whose heads had been injured in a definite locality (and who presented symptoms corresponding to those described by me), but who had no recollection of the injury. An examination of the head might have revealed the fact, and the symptoms would have confirmed the particular locality; but the physician, being a follower of the Freudian school, preferred to psycho-analyse the patients in order to get a confession of their history from their subconscious minds, and, having ascertained the previous injury in this manner, and its seat, they were then surgically treated. Surely this is a roundabout way of getting at the facts of a case. The following is the literal report, taken from the *British Medical Journal*, March 11, 1922:

Reports of Societies

Psychological Analysis in Diagnosis

At a meeting of the Medico-Psychological Association of Great Britain and Ireland, held in the rooms of the Medical Society of London, on February 23rd, with the President, Dr. C. Hubert Bond, in the Chair, Dr. T. S. Good (Ashurst Hospital, Oxford) read a paper on the use of analysis in diagnosis. Analysis, he said, must be used by every practising physician and surgeon in all kinds of cases; and they must be influenced in their decision by what they saw, felt, and heard. Until a quite recent date, the material upon which the doctor drew had been the conscious only; but, thanks to the ingenuity, the genius, and the patient work of Freud, a new source of medical knowledge had been opened to the profession, for he found that the solution of many of the problems as to the cause of neuroses and psychoses lay deeply buried in the unconscious mind of the patient. By special methods of technique, these elements could be disclosed and brought into consciousness, and energy, hitherto dammed back, could be released to bring about improvement or cure. This had never been better demonstrated than during and after the war, in cases of shell shock and neurasthenia; for many cases had been cured by psychotherapy, of which psycho-analysis was one of the instruments. By following the method of free association, physical conditions could be diagnosed which would, otherwise, escape notice, or be only partially understood, because the key to the solution of the physical mischief lay repressed in the unconscious, and so could not be furnished by the patient, in response to the usual examination.

Dr. Good elaborated the point by quoting, in detail, two cases, which had been diagnosed, respectively, as neurasthenia and hysteria.

The *first* case was that of a man, aged 50, who, after four years of war, was invalided out in 1918, with the diagnosis of neurasthenia. He had been under a varied treatment, and had tried, but with only partial success, to resume his pre-war occupation of motor-body making. There was nothing abnormal in the family history. At his first attendance at the clinic he was obviously *apathetic and depressed*, questions being answered slowly, and with apparent indifference. He complained of a headache, great depression, inability to work, loss of memory, and was puzzled as to what could be the matter with him. He said that, at times, he felt "lost and giddy". The right side of his face did not move so well as the left. The tongue was protruded straight; the pupils were normal, and equal in their reactions; fundi and vision were also normal. The only abnormality in the reflexes was that the plantar, on the right, was indefinite. Oppenheim's reflex was absent. Sensation, co-ordination, muscular sense, were normal; also muscle tone, and there appeared to be nothing wrong with the organs; the pulse rate was 80.

The two abnormalities mentioned indicated that the case was not purely functional; but they did not form a sufficient basis for a firm diagnosis. He was unable to remember a certain period of his war experiences; he showed a disinclination to talk of the war, beyond stating that to it he attributed all his disability; *he had a desire to be quietly by himself.* After the third interview, the man's demeanour changed. and he began to co-operate in his treatment, and to associate, with the result that his thoughts and feelings on his illness became clearer. A part of his life which he could not account for, however, was a period during a voyage at sea. He was on a ship when it was torpedoed at sea; but he could remember nothing between that explosion and his being in hospital. But details emerged in his mind, as he evinced more interest and showed co-operation, and eventually he was able to describe what happened after the ship was struck. It appears that he was thrown across the cabin, and his head came into violent contact with a bulkhead, *injuring his left parietal region*; he remembered feeling and hearing his skull crack. Feeling very sick and ill, he rushed, with others, on to the deck. He was rescued from the sea, and taken to hospital. The whole of this amnesia was removed at one sitting, and the patient then expressed great surprise, remarking, "I do not know why it is, but I feel all right, and am glad I can now remember everything." On returning to the clinic, a fortnight later, he said his memory was good, and he felt better; but, instead of the dull headache, he now had a new, and a more acute pain in the head, such as he had never experienced before, except when his head struck the ship's bulkhead, and the site was the same. This directed attention to a probable *injury of the left parietal region*, perhaps a fracture, with some resultant injury of the brain.

A surgeon thereupon operated, and discovered a 2-in. fracture at the exact site of the pain, and some bruising of brain substance. Previously there had been no suspicion of an organic element in the case. In this case, the amnesia having been cured, the clue was supplied by the patient himself. His attention to that stage had been so concentrated on his mental feelings, that physical sensations were unnoticed until the mental conflict had been solved. The man had now recovered his mental poise; but the pain in the head was still present, and, following the operation, he had slight hemiplegia.

The *second* case was that of a man, aged 25, reputed normal before the war. After serving two years in the army, he was discharged, the diagnosis being "*hysterical fits*". When his mother brought him to the clinic, she said his disposition had now completely altered, for, at times, he was *violent, aggressive, and irritable.* He was said to have been having two kinds of fits; but both were ushered in by *twitching* on the right side of the face. Sometimes he became rigid, and seemed dazed and dull afterwards, with headache. In the other kind of fits he threw himself about, and was afterwards violent and irritable. The man was unable to remember any of the fits. When pressed to talk about the war, he became irritable. Generally the reflexes on the right side were greater than on the left; on the right, also, there was some muscular weakness. At the second interview he was induced to talk about the war, when it was found that his memory of events for long periods was very defective; he did not remember why he had been sent home, nor when the fits started.

The detailed history, which Dr. Good read, showed that his trouble was connected with heavy trench-mortar warfare, in which he received *a severe head injury.* By the method of association, the blank interval was made good, and then the patient talked freely about the episodes he experienced. After the recovery of the memory, *the emotional fits ceased, but the rigid fits* increased in frequency. The right-sided weakness seemed to indicate that, on that side, there was increased intracranial pressure; probably due to head injury. Later, *the operation of decompression was performed*; and, since then, he had only two epileptiform attacks. He was discharged three months later. Four weeks afterwards his mother brought him again, and said there had been no attacks since he was discharged, and that he was now working as a gardener.

After pointing out the parallelism in the two cases, Dr. Good commented on the fact that one of them reacted by being depressed (introverted); the other by becoming excited (extroverted). The cases showed that psycho-analysis could be of use in diagnosing organic condition.

The President, in thanking Dr. Good for his interesting contribution, deprecated any tendency to regard the materialistic and the psychiatric schools, or lines of thought, as being opposed to each other. The cases described in the paper showed how useful was the broad, inclusive view, in unravelling difficult cases.

A short discussion followed, and, in his reply, Dr. Good elaborated at greater length some of the aspects of this line of inquiry.

It will be noticed that *the first case is absolutely identical with my cases of melancholic depression*, due to lesions in the parietal region, of which a list of about 300 cases has been given in this chapter; and *the other corresponds with my cases of irritability, violence, and convulsive fits due to lesions of the temporal region* (see next chapter). In the latter case, however, Dr. Good, as is so often the case, omitted to state the site of the lesion, as if it were of no importance which part of the head was affected. It is also significant that these cases were diagnosed as "neurasthenic" and "hysterical", which helps to explain why so many physicians believe that head injuries are never, or hardly ever, followed by mental derangement.

In all cases of head injury it is very important to detect the malingerer, especially in cases of mental depression. If the symptoms correspond with the effects of a particular brain-lesion, this will help the physician in the diagnosis. For example, L. W. WEBER (*Deutsche Mediz. Wochenschrift*, 1905) was consulted about a man, 32 years of age, who had injured his occipital bone in a fall on the head, and was accused of simulation. Dr. Weber diagnosed genuine melancholia by the nature of the symptoms and the seat of the lesion.

CHAPTER VII

IRASCIBILITY IN LESIONS OF THE LOWER PART OF THE TEMPORAL LOBES

It will be seen from several hundred examples cited in the following pages that, when the *base of the temporal* lobes is stimulated, states of excitement (irascibility) are produced, ranging from the simple form of anger to furious, and even homicidal, mania.

Anger is a primitive emotion, and has, for its object, the overcoming of obstacles and foes, for the purpose of self-preservation. By increasing the bodily energy, anger enables us to remove things that threaten us, and is, thus, a reflex mechanism of immense value in the struggle for existence. It is an innate mechanism, manifested long before the living creature has had any experience. The disposition to it varies in degree, in different individuals. In its healthy state, it gives executive power; in its morbid state, it is manifested in chronic bad temper and quarrelsomeness. Its extreme can be observed in "irascible insanity" (acute mania), in which there are ungovernable spontaneous motor impulses and violent anger; generally without loss of knowledge of the surroundings. The person may be so furious as to exhaust himself in shouts, threats, and actions; or the passions may be less vehement, but in all cases it is "anger". *The evidence that the temporal lobe is in some way the centre of a reflex mechanism for the protection of self, by producing states of excitement which give additional energy to the entire body, is overwhelming.*

N. C. Paulesco (*Arch. Internat. de Physiologie*, 1922) admitted that the instinct of self-defence must have a centre in the cortex of the brain; a conclusion at which he arrived as the result of his experiments on animals.

When FERRIER stimulated the lower temporal region in cats and jackals, "the application of the electrodes in this region caused the animal to make a sudden spring, or bound forward, pricking up both ears as if preparing to *fight*, and opening of the mouth associated with vocalisation, and other signs of emotional expression, such as spitting, and lashing the tail as if in *rage*" (op. cit.).

EXAMPLES OF LESIONS OF THE BASE OF THE TEMPORAL LOBES, FOLLOWED BY IRASCIBILITY, IMPULSIVENESS, AND HOMICIDAL MANIA

I. *Surgical Treatment of Injuries of Temporal Lobes Resulting in Recovery*

H. A. Powell.	Surg. Aspect of Traumatic Insanity, 1893. *Manslaughter.*
Jas. Howden.	Journal of Mental Science, 1875. *Homicidal.*
W. S. Savory.	British Medical Journal, 1869.
Lamphear.	University Medical Magazine, 1893. *Homicidal.*
Ernest Laplace.	Medical and Surgical Reporter, 1896.
Chas. Gibbs.	International Clinics, 1902.
Sir Thomas Smith.	Lancet, 1879. *Bullet wound.*
John. J. Waddelow.	Ibidem, 1922. *Dangerous lunatic.*
Francis Skae.	Edinburgh Med. Journ., Vol. XI. Case 3. Seven years after injury.
W. B. Fletcher.	American Journ. of Insanity, 1887. *Epilepsy cured.* Twenty-four years after injury.
E. v. Bergmann.	Volkmann's Hefte, No. 190.
E. Hoffmann.	Deutsche Medizinische Wochenschrift, 1881.
E. Sommer.	Casuistik der Gehirnverletzungen, 1874.
P. Guder.	Geistesstörungen nach Kopfverletzungen, 1886.
Serger.	Allg. Zeitschrift f. Psychiatrie, 1911.
G. Burkhardt.	Ibidem, 1891. *Homicidal.*

H. F. W. Wendt.	Ibidem, 1875. *Bullet wound.* Five years after injury.
Schupfer.	Monatsschrift f. Psychiatrie, 1908.
M. Astrazaturow.	Ibidem, 1911. *A series of cases.*
A. Spanbock.	Neurologisches Centralblatt, 1895.
R. v. Krafft-Ebing.	Über d.d. Geh. u. Kpfverl. herv. psych. Krankh., 1868.
D. Mollière.	Lyon Médicale. 1881. *Acute mania.*
Boubila & Pantaloni.	Gazette des Hôpitaux, 1892. *Epilepsy cured.* Twenty-five years after injury.
Eugène Azam.	Arch. Génér. de Médecine, 1881. *Bullet wound.* Eleven years after injury.
J. A. E. Estlander.	Finiska Lak Handlingar, 1897.
Cohuirsco & Milhaerco.	Spitalerd, 1907. *Acute mania.*
Wm. Sharpe.	Diagn. and Treatm. of Brain Injuries, 1920. *Mania and Epilepsy. Recovery after removal of tumour.*

II. *Examples of Cases of Temporal Injuries, not Surgically Treated; most of them with post-mortem evidence of haemorrhage into middle fossae*

J. Russell.	British Medical Journal, 1865.
Reginald Harrison.	Ibidem, 1869.
W. S. Savory.	Ibidem, 1869.
J. Lane.	Ibidem, 1872.
Shaw & Cripps.	Ibidem, 1890.
W. H. Battle.	Ibidem, 1890.
E. Tredinnick.	Ibidem, 1900. *Two cases. One acute mania; one homicide.*
Lawson & Major.	Lancet, 1876. *Depressed temp. bone. Acute mania.*
N. H. Alcock.	Ibidem, 1877.
James Ross.	Dis. of the Nerv. Syst., 1883. *Several cases.*
W. J. Mickle.	Journal of Mental Science, 1881. *Homicide.*
W. J. Mickle.	Ibidem, 1885. *Homicide.*
J. R. Whitwell.	Ibidem, 1891.

B. B. Fox.	Ibidem, 1891.
T. Claye Shaw.	Archives of Medicine, 1882.
G. J. Guthrie.	"Injuries to Head, affecting the Brain."
G. Thompson.	Brain, 1894.
Francis Skae.	Edinburgh Medical Journal, 1866. *Developed epilepsy.*
Chas. L. Dana.	Journal of Nerv. and Ment. Dis., 1889.
R. W. Amidon.	Ibidem, 1880. *Bullet wound.*
M. Jowett.	Western Journ. of Med., 1868. *Aphasic but swearing.*
Chas. Phelps.	New York Medical Journal. 1893. *Forty-two cases.*
Daniel Clarke.	American Journal of Insanity, 1881.
J. B. Andrews.	Ibidem, Vol. XXV.
T. Kirkbride.	Ibidem, 1879.
R. v. Krafft-Ebing.	Op. cit., 1868. *Three medico-legal cases of homicide.*
R. v. Krafft-Ebing.	Friedreich's Blätter, 1868. *Several cases.*
G. Spies.	Casuistik d. traum. Manie, 1869. *Homicide.*
Serger.	Allg. Zeitschr. f. Psychiatrie, 1911. *Homicide.*
A. Eichholt.	Ibidem, 1885.
E. Kundt.	Ibidem, 1894. *Three cases.*
F. Meschede.	Ibidem, 1873. *Two cases of epilepsy and homicide.*
T. Krebs.	Ibidem, 1895.
H. Voppel.	Ibidem, Vol. XIV. *Two cases.*
Stuckle.	Ibidem, Vol. XIII. *Developed epilepsy. Medico-legal case.*
C. F. Flemming.	Ibidem, Vol. IX.
J. Wagner.	Jahrbuch f. Psychiatrie, 1884.
A. Hartmann.	Archiv. f. Psychiatrie, 1884. *Several cases.*
Lieber & Bedstübner.	Ibidem, Vol. XV.
Ludwig Meyer.	Ibidem, 1872. *Epilepsy.*
E. K. Hoffmann.	Vierteljahrschr. f. Psychiatrie, Vol. II.
Max Huppert.	Archiv. d. Heilkunde, 1875. *Acute mania and epilepsy.*

C. A. T. Billroth.	Chirurgische Klinik, 1871.
A. Pick.	Prager med. Wochenschrift, 1880.
F. L. A. Kelp.	Deutsches Archiv. f. Klin. Medizin. 1872.
H. T. Tiling.	St. Petersburger med. Wochenschrift, 1879.
E. Schäfer.	Centralblatt f. Nervenheilkunde, 1881.
Erich Feuchtwanger.	Funktionen d. Stirnhirns, 1922. *Several cases.*
Paul Schüller.	Psychosen n. Kopfverletzungen, 1882. *Several cases.*
Bernhard Beck.	Die Schädelverletzungen, 1865. *Several cases.*
Landerer & Lutz.	Christophsbad Asyl. Berichte, 1878. *Several cases.*
L. Schlager.	Zeitschr. d. Ges. d. Aerzte z. Wien. Vol. VII and VIII. *Several cases.*
Bax.	Fricke's Zeitschrift, Vol. VIII.
H. Demme.	Milit.-Chir. Studien, 1864. *Several cases of bullet wounds.*
R. Bruggia.	Arch. Ital. par la Malat. Nerv., 1884. *Aphasic, but swearing.*
J. Christian.	Archiv. de Neurologie, 1889. *Bullet wound.*
F. Lallemand.	Réch. Anat.-Path. sur l'Encéphale.
L. F. Arnaud.	L'Encéphale, 1888.
O. Herpin.	Progrès Médical, 1876. *Several cases.*
Julien Tellier.	Traumatismes du Crâne, 1890.
M. A. Foville.	Annales Médico-Psychologiques, 1871.

Recently several observers have confirmed my observation that *tumours*, situated in this region, may give rise to convulsive fits in over 50 per cent. of all recorded cases. FOSTER KENNEDY, *Arch. of International Medicine*, 1911 (in all but two of his cases), and THEODOR MEYNERT, long ago, found that in epilepsy the greatest atrophy and loss of weight is in the temporal lobes; but that is all that has been acknowledged so far. For a time it has been thought that excitation of the motor area gave rise to epilepsy; but it does so only in what is called Jacksonian epilepsy, not in genuine epilepsy. Epileptic fits caused by disturbances in the temporal lobes can be distinguished from other forms of epilepsy by the frequency of some warning or "aura" previous to the attack. Among the following will be found a large number of cases of violent mania, which also developed convulsive fits.

III. *Examples of Cases of Tumours of Temporal Lobes with Symptoms of Violent Mania*

W. Boyd & S. Hopwood.	Brain and Lancet, 1913. *Chronic mania.*
Jas. Crichton-Browne.	British Medical Journal, 1873.
W. T. Gairdner.	Ibidem, 1873.
W. T. Gairdner.	Ibidem, 1877. *Mistaken for hysteria.*
A. Hughes Bennett.	Brain. 1878.
Wm. Gowers.	Ibidem, 1910.
Alexander Bruce.	Ibidem, 1883. *Mistaken for hysteria.*
Frederic Bateman.	On "Aphasia", 1890. *Developed epilepsy and mania.*
T. S. Clouston.	Journal of Mental Science, 1872. *Developed epilepsy and mania.*
T. S. Clouston.	Ibidem, 1875. *Developed epilepsy and mania. Two cases.*
W. H. Packer.	Ibidem, 1882.
B. M. MacDowall.	Ibidem, 1881. *Homicidal.*
J. Rorie.	Ibidem, 1890. *Homicidal.*
Conolly Norman.	Ibidem, 1890. *Homicidal.*
Conolly Norman.	Ibidem, 1893.
W. J. A. Erskine.	Ibidem, 1901.
J. A. Arbuckle.	Glasgow Medical Journal, 1876.
Samuel Wilks.	Guy's Hospital Reports, 1866.
B. Ball.	Buffalo Medical Journal, 1898. *Mistaken for hysteria.*
J. Russell.	Medical Times and Gazette, 1873. *Mania and epilepsy.*

S. J. Sharkey.	Journal of Nerv. and Ment. Dis., 1889. *Homicidal.*
Mills & McConnell.	Ibidem, 1895. *Homicidal.*
F. X. Dercum.	Ibidem, 1912.
J. B. Prowbridge.	Ibidem. 1891. *Epilepsy and mania.*
H. M. Hurd.	American Journal of Insanity, 1896.
A. Gordon.	Medical Journal and Record, 1926.
Leonardo Bianchi.	The Mechanism of the Brain. *Mania and epilepsy.*
H. Vogt.	"Epilepsie im Kindesalter", 1910. *Three cases.*
F. Meschede.	Allg. Zeitschr. f. Psychiatrie, 1873. *Two cases.*
Otto Snell.	Ibidem. 1875.
Stuckle.	Ibidem, Vol. XIII. *Developed epilepsy and mania.*
A. Richter.	Ibidem, 1883.
Zohreb.	Ibidem, 1886. *Developed epilepsy and mania.*
J. Jensen.	Ibidem, 1889.
W. Fränkel.	Ibidem, 1896.
Kaplan.	Ibidem, 1897. *Acute mania.*
B. Pfeifer.	Ibidem, 1910. Case 32. *Acute mania.*
Liebscher.	Prager med. Wochenschrift, 1906.
E. Klebs.	Prager Vierteljahrschrift, 1877. *Acute mania.*
Lindström.	Hygiea, Vol. XVIII. *Acute mania.*
H. Schüle.	Sektionserg. b. Geisteskranken, 1874. *Acute mania.*
Jacob Weiss.	Wiener med. Wochenschrift, 1877. *Acute mania.*
E. K. Hoffmann.	Zeitschr. f. rationelle Medizin, 1869.
H. Oppenheim.	Archiv. f. Psychiatrie, 1877.
I. S. Steiner.	Ibidem, 1910.
M. Huppert.	Archiv. der Heilkunde, 1875.
H. Lutz.	Bayr. Aerztl. Intelligenzblatt, 1864.
C. Bauze.	Jahrbuch f. Kinderheilkunde, 1876.
Brault & Loeper.	Arch. Gén. de Médicine, 1900. *Mistaken for hysteria.*

N. Rousseau.	L'Encéphale, 1888. *Two cases.*
N. Chambard.	Ibidem, 1881.
Geoffrey.	Annales Médico-Psychologiques, 1865.
C. Bouchet.	Ibidem, 1853.
B. Ball.	Ibidem, 1876.
P. Rey.	Ibidem, 1882.
B. M. MacDowall.	Rivista di Freniatria, 1889. *Homicidal and epileptic.*

IV. *Examples of Cases of Inflammation and Softening of Temporal Lobes*

Byrom Bramwell.	Edinburgh Medical Journal, 1879. *Homicidal.*
R. B. Mitchell.	Ibidem, 1883. *Homicidal.*
T. R. Glynn.	British Medical Journal, 1878. *Homicidal.*
W. Boyd & S. Hopwood.	Lancet, 1913. *Homicidal.*
T. Crisp English.	Ibidem, 1904. *Developed epilepsy and homicidal mania.*
Lauder Lindsay.	Murray's Royal Asylum Report, 1860. *Homicidal.*
Kenneth McLeod.	Journal of Mental Science, 1861. *Homicidal.*
J. MacKenzie Bacon.	Ibidem, 1869.
S. W. D. Williams.	Ibidem, 1869. *Developed epilepsy and homicidal mania.*
F. Needham.	Ibidem, 1872. *Homicidal.*
T. S. Clouston.	Ibidem, 1875. *Developed epilepsy and homicidal mania.*
T. B. Worthington.	Ibidem, 1880.
Wm. Julius Mickle.	Ibidem, 1880. *Four cases.*
Wm. Julius Mickle.	Ibidem, 1881. *Developed epilepsy and homicidal mania.*
W. R. Wood.	Ibidem, 1884. *Developed epilepsy and homicidal mania.*
Frank Hay.	Ibidem, 1895. *Developed epilepsy and homicidal mania.*

PLATE XV

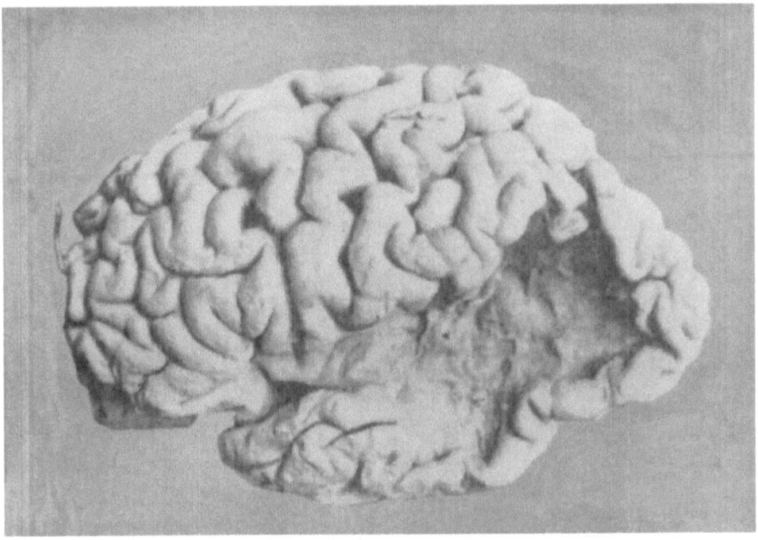

SOFTENING OF TEMPORAL LOBE IN ACUTE MANIA

(*See page* 136)

Plate XVI

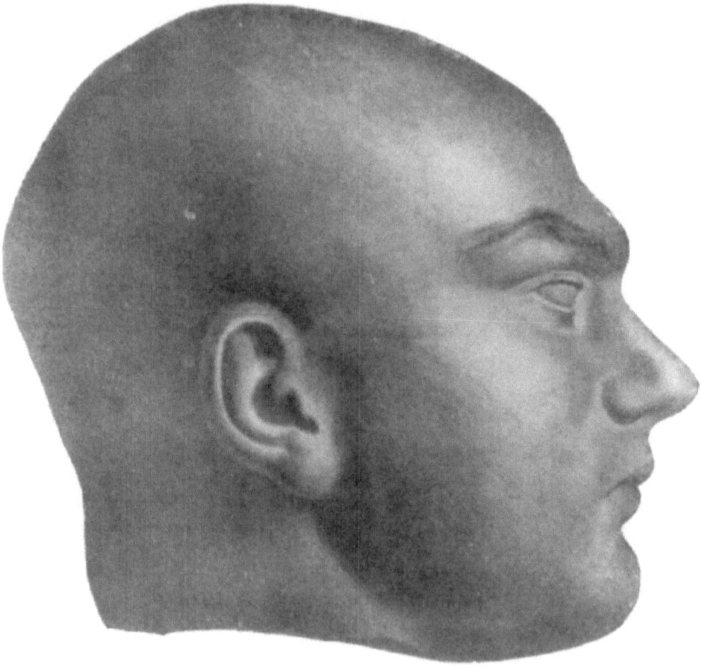

CAST OF HEAD OF A PARRICIDE
Large in the temporal region (*see page* 258)

T. S. Bolton.	Ibidem, 1905. *Developed epilepsy and homicidal mania.*
G. H. Savage.	Brain, 1879. *Homicidal.*
Samuel Wilks.	Guy's Hospital Reports, 1866. *Epilepsy and homicidal mania.*
Samuel Wilks.	Guy's Hospital Reports, 1881. *Epilepsy and homicidal mania.*
T. D. Greenlees.	Amer. Journ. of Insanity, 1887. *Two cases of homicide.*
Adolf Meyer.	Ibidem, 1895. *Homicide.*
Bancroft.	Ibidem, 1879. *With sensory aphasia.*
W. L. Worcester.	Ibidem, 1896.
J. B. Prowbridge.	Journal of Nerv. and Ment. Dis., 1891. *Homicidal.*
A. M. Barrett.	Ibidem, 1910.
Chas. L. Dana.	Ibidem, 1889.
Mills & McConnell.	Ibidem, 1895. *Homicidal with sensory aphasia.*
Bleynie.	Diss. sur l'Inflamm. du Cerveau. *Homicidal.*
Anglade.	Gazette Méd. de Bordeaux, 1911. *Homicidal.*
F. Baizer.	Gazette Médicale de Paris, 1884. *With sensory aphasia.*
J. Luys.	L'Encéphale, 1891.
Labori.	Bull. de la Soc. Anatom., 1867. *Homicidal.*
J. Christian.	Annales Médico-Psychologiques, 1874. *Homicidal.*
Clovis Gallopin.	Ibidem, 1879.
M. A. Foville.	Ibidem, 1882. *Developed epilepsy and homicidal mania.*
A. Cullère.	Ibidem, 1890.
C. Bouchet.	De l'Epilepsie. *Several cases.*
Bourneville & D'Ollier.	Recherches s. l'Epilepsie, 1881. *Two cases.*
M. Mariani.	Archiv. Ital. par le mal. nerv., 1886. *Homicidal.*
Leonardo Bianchi.	Mechanism of the Brain, 1922. Case 9.
Leonardo Bianchi.	La Emiplegia. *With sensory aphasia.*

A. Tamburini.	Rivista Sper. di Freniatria, Vol. V. *Developed epilepsy.*
G. Seppilli.	Rivista Sper. di Freniatria. 1884. *With sensory aphasia.*
H. Liepman.	Neur. Centralblatt, 1900. *Homicidal. Sensory aphasia.*
Leop. Lacquer.	Ibidem, 1888. *Homicidal. Sensory aphasia.*
Schäfer.	Centralblatt f. Nervenheilkunde, 1881. *Homicidal. Sensory aphasia.*
M. Bernhardt.	Ibidem, 1882. *Homicidal. Sensory aphasia.*
Albert Rosenthal.	Ibidem, 1886. *Two cases. Homicidal. Sensory aphasia.*
Albert Rosenthal.	Ibidem, 1884. *Homicidal.*
Albert Rosenthal.	Ibidem, 1889. *Homicidal.*
Rasori,	Ibidem, Vol. XIV. *Homicidal.*
H. Zingerle.	Journ. f. Psych. u. Neurologie, 1911. *Homicidal.*
H. Lutz.	Bayr. Aerztl. Intelligenzblatt, 1864. *Homicidal.*
O. Körner.	Berliner Klin. Wochenschrift, 1885. *Homicidal.*
Adolf Kussmaul.	Ibidem, 1885. *Whole temp. lobe destroyed without sensory aphasia.*
G. H. Bergmann.	Allg. Zeitschr. f. Psychiatrie, Vol. III.
Stuckle.	Ibidem, Vol. XIII. *Homicidal.*
H. Voppel.	Ibidem, Vol. XIV. *Homicidal.*
Feith.	Ibidem, 1867. *Developed epilepsy and homicidal mania.*
C. Fröhlich.	Ibidem, 1875. *Two cases of homicidal mania.*
L. Bruns.	Ibidem, 1892. *With sensory aphasia.*
O. Hebold.	Ibidem, 1894. *With sensory aphasia.*
L. Willé.	Ibidem, 1875. *Homicidal.*
Otto Snell.	Ibidem, 1875. *Developed epilepsy and homicidal mania.*
Zohreb.	Ibidem, 1896.
B. Ascher.	Ibidem, 1893.

F. Lührmann.	Ibidem, 1896. *Developed epilepsy and homicidal mania.*
H. Schüle.	Sektionserg. b. Geisteskranken, 1874. *Three cases with sensory aphasia.*
B. Beck.	Archiv. f. Psychiatrie, Vol. XV. *Developed epilepsy and homicidal mania.*
Ludwig Meyer.	Ibidem, 1872. *Developed epilepsy and homicidal mania.*
Fürstner & Stühlinger.	Ibidem, 1886. *Developed epilepsy and homicidal mania.*
Th. Zacher.	Ibidem, 1888. *Homicidal.*
M. Köppen.	Ibidem, 1896. *Homicidal.*
A. Alzheimer.	Ibidem, 1897. *Homicidal.*
A. Pick.	Ibidem, 1892. *With sensory aphasia.*
W. Bischoff.	Ibidem, 1889. *With sensory aphasia. Three cases.*
J. Fritsch.	Wiener Medizinische Presse, 1879. *With sensory aphasia.*

It will be noticed that among the cases quoted there are a number in which sensory aphasia (word-deafness) occurred. Altogether, I have noted that sensory aphasia and acute mania may occur together in lesions of the temporal lobes; whereas word-blindness is never associated with it, but occasionally with melancholia in lesions of the parietal lobes.

In the *Gazette Médicale de Bordeaux*, July 16, 1911, is an article entitled "La jargonaphasie logorrhéique", in which volubility without word-deafness in lesions of Wernicke's area is described. When the lesion bordered on the parietal, the patients were sad, otherwise all the cases were gay and *irascible.*

Sometimes the temporal lobes are sound; but distension of the lateral ventricles has given rise to pressure on them. Sometimes, as I have seen in three cases following motor-car smashes, mania and epilepsy are caused by fractures of the base of the skull, through extravasation of blood into the brain tissues, and tearing of the structure of this region. Maniacal symptoms may, also, be the result of pressure caused by tumours in the neighbourhood, such as tumours of the hypophysis. SCHUSTER, in his work on *Brain Tumours*, mentions eleven cases of this kind, followed by violent mania.

V. *Other Examples of Subcortical Tumours Causing Oedema of Temporal Lobes and followed by Mania*

W. B. Ransome.	Brain, 1895.
A. H. Martin.	British Medical Journal, 1875.
James Collier.	Ibidem, 1924. *Three cases.*
N. Friedreich.	Intracranial Tumours, 1853.
F. K. Stahl.	Allg. Zeitschrift f. Psychiatrie, 1869–73. *Six cases.*
Gottfried Jehn.	Archiv. f. Psychiatrie, 1878. *Three cases.*
C. Fürstner.	Ibidem, 1875.
A. Holländer.	Jahrbücher d. Psychiatrie, Vol. III.
M. Rosenthal.	Med. Jahrb. d. Ges. d. Aerzte z. Wien, 1882.
J. B. Falret.	Bull. de la Société Anat. de Paris, 1866.

If this theory be correct, one would also expect to find in chronic mania an increase in the size of the temporal lobes. Indeed, I have seen actual swellings of the temporal bones above the ears, but such conditions are usually not taken noti ce of.

VI. *Examples of Cases of Abnormal Development of the Temporal Lobes with Symptoms of Homicidal Mania*

H. Voppel.	Allg. Zeitschr. f. Psychiatrie, Vol. XIV. *Several cases.*
Arnold Pick.	Prager Medizin. Wochenschrift, 1879. *Homicidal.*
Warren L. Babcock.	State Hospitals' Bulletin, 1896.

Experts will be interested in the large percentage of *homicidal* cases in *inflammatory* lesions of the temporal lobes, and—as I have already mentioned—the frequency of *epileptic* fits in the case of *tumours* of the same area. I called attention to these symptoms in temporal lesions as long ago as 1901 (in my book on *The Mental Functions of the Brain*); but it is only within the last few years that various observers have confirmed this observation. Its importance is shown by the following two interesting cases.

The first one is that reported in the daily newspapers of October 6, 1927. An ex-soldier, an inmate of the Knowle Mental Hospital, had committed suicide, and at the inquest the following facts became known. Two years previously, this young man had been sentenced to eighteen months' imprisonment for attempting to strangle someone in a train, and the judge then said that "if the accused had not been wounded in the war, he would have been ordered a flogging". After three weeks' imprisonment, he was certified a criminal lunatic, and transferred to Knowle Institution, where it was found that a piece of shrapnel, in the *temporal* region of his brain, caused him to have attacks of confusion resembling epilepsy.

The second case is that of Perry (reported in *The Times* of June 24, 1919), who murdered a family at Forest Gate, with comprehensive and aimless brutality, which would lead one to suspect mental disorder. Evidence was given that the side of his head had been injured, and was painful at the spot, that he was subject to hallucinations of hearing, and had epileptic fits, though some years back: that he came of an insane stock; that one of his sisters was an epileptic; and that he had consulted a doctor about his condition prior to the murder.

One of the medical witnesses acknowledged that he would have recommended an operation on the injured area of the man's skull. Still, the jury found the prisoner guilty, and he was sentenced to death. The Lord Chief Justice, on appeal, pointed out that the crux of the case was whether there was evidence that, at the time when the murders were committed, the murderer was suffering from an epileptic attack; otherwise, it would be dangerous if a man were to say: "I once had an epileptic fit, and everything that happens thereafter must be put down to that." The appeal was dismissed, and Perry was hanged.

The temporal lobes are separated from the internal ear by a very thin partition of bone, and can, therefore, be irritated by *middle ear affections*, or the disease may actually extend to them; in both events, leading to various degrees of excitement and even acute mania—symptoms which disappear with the treatment of the originating cause. Affections of hearing differ, in this respect, from affections of sight, which, when due to central lesion, lead to mental depression, paroxysms of fear and melancholia, and, sometimes, attempts at self-destruction.

I have also observed that, while the discharge from the ear continues, the patient may be quiet; but that, on cessation of the escape of pus, a violent attack of mania may ensue. Not all these facts are yet confirmed; but similar observations have been made by a number of authors:—Griesinger, Schüle, Jacobi, Köppe, Körner, Huguenin, Morel, Paul Robin, Bennett, and MacEwen, besides those whose cases will be quoted.

VII. *Examples of Chronic Middle Ear Disease with Symptoms of Homicidal Mania*

Wm. MacCormac.	Lancet, 1886.
W. Sohier Bryant.	Journal of Nerv. and Mental Dis., 1906. *Several cases.*
Medico-Legal Case.	American Journal of Insanity, Vol. V, p. 34.
E. Grissom.	Ibidem, 1877.
G. C. Bablett.	Ibidem, 1877. *Two cases.*

W. H. Bennett.	Dublin Quarterly Journal of Medical Science, 1871.
K. Cramer.	Gerichtliche Psychiatrie. *Murdered her children.*
H. Spitta.	Prakt. Beitr. z. ger. aerztl. Psychologie. *Medico-legal case of homicide.*
Jansen.	Berliner Klinische Wochenschrift, 1891.
L. Schlager.	Zeitschr. d. Ges. d. Aerzte z. Wien, Vol. XIII.
Homer.	Monatsschrift f. Ohrenheilkunde, 1863.
H. Schüle.	Handbuch d. Geisteskrankheiten, 1878. *Three cases.*
E. Bouchut.	Gazette des Hôpitaux, 1877.
H. Kukarzewski.	Progrès Médical, 1894.
A. Babinsky.	Larguedoc Médical, 1891.
G. Fabri.	Italia Medica, 1883.
Edwin W. Day.	Annals of Otology, 1911. *Two cases.*

VIII. *Examples of Cases of Middle Ear Disease Recovering After Surgical Treatment*

W. Rhys Williams.	Lancet, 1877.
Watson Cheyne.	British Medical Journal, 1890.
Francis Skae.	Edinburgh Medical Journal, Vol. XI.
G. C. Bablett.	American Journal of Insanity, 1877. *Two cases.*
J. O. Green.	Boston Medical and Surgical Journal, 1890.
W. S. Bryant.	Journal of Nerv. and Mental Disease, 1906.
Ludwig Meyer.	Deutsche Klinik, Vol. VII.
J. M. Köppe.	Archiv. f. Ohrenheilkunde, 1875. *Homicidal.*
H. Schüle.	Handbuch der Geisteskrankheiten, 1872. *Three cases.*
E. Bouchut.	Gazette des Hôpitaux, 1877.
B. Ball.	L'Encéphale, 1881. Five years after a blow on left ear.
R. v. Krafft-Ebing.	Op. cit., 1868. *Violent and destructive.*

That ear disease, irritating, or extending to, the temporal

lobes, may not only cause mania, but also fits, was already known to J. A. ORMEROD (*Brain*, 1884), who found, among 100 cases of epilepsy, 46 suffering from ear disease; also to P. MACBRIDE (*Edinburgh Medical Journal*, 1880). W. SOHIER BRYANT had an article in the *Journal of Nervous and Mental Disease*, 1906, on "The Great Psychical Importance of Ear Disease", in which he gave numerous examples of purulent inflammation of the middle ear, followed by psychoses, which disappeared on treatment of the ear trouble. GEOFFREY W. ROBINSON (*Journal of Neurology and Psychopathology*, 1927) examined 200 certified insane people, and found 66 per cent. of the total number to be suffering from aural disease.

If further proof were needed of the fact that congestion of the temporal lobes leads to irascibility, and tendencies to violence and destruction, we have it in the frequency of *haematomata auris*, which seem to be due to a sanguineous perichondrial effusion of the auricle, and appear to withdraw the blood from the adjacent brain substance; consequently, on the appearance of the haematoma, it is not uncommon to find that the mania ceases.

IX. *Examples of Cases of Haematoma Auris in Violent Mania, Recovery after Treatment*

Teats.	British Medical Journal, 1881. *Homicidal.*
Fred. Needham.	Ibidem, 1890.
Tishkoff.	Lancet, 1892.
E. H. van Deusen.	American Journal of Insanity, 1874.
P. W. MacDonald.	Ibidem, 1887.

Neurologists and alienists should, also, be interested in the fact that in the congestion of the temporal lobes caused by various lesions, *patients otherwise aphasic* can still utter "oaths" when they can articulate nothing else. Sir W. T. GAIRDNER

PLATE XVII

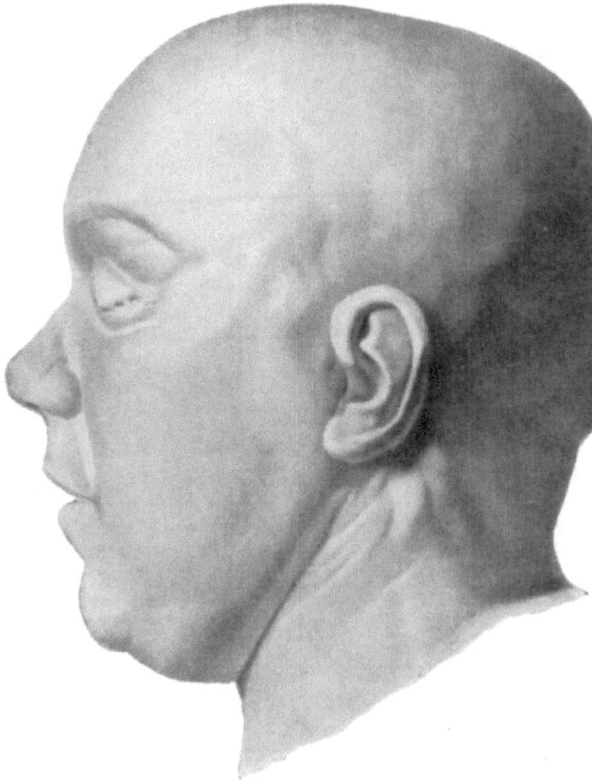

DR. WILLIAM PALMER, MURDERER

The head is large in the posterior temporal area

Plate XVIII

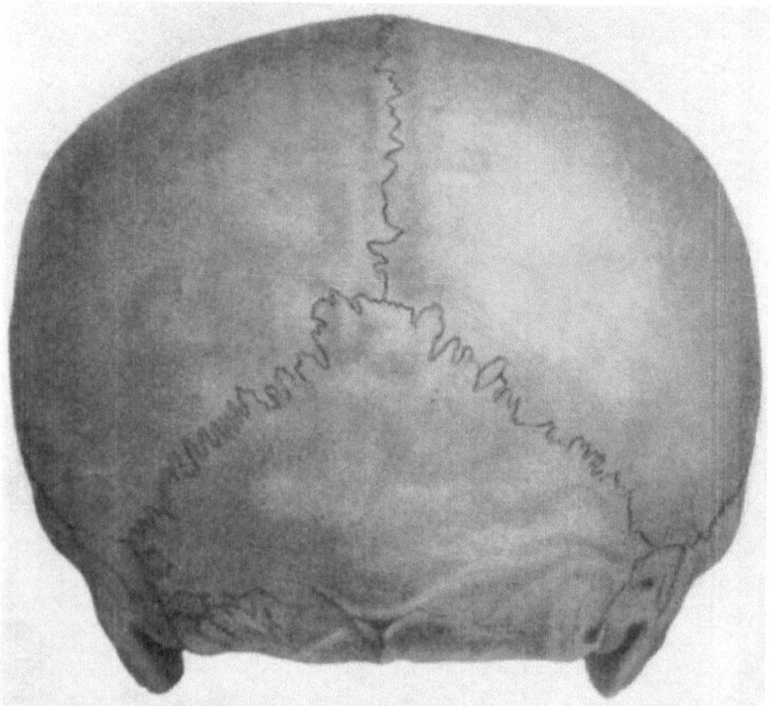

SKULL OF A HOMICIDAL CRIMINAL
Notice extraordinary width of head

and HUGHLINGS JACKSON called attention to this particular affection, and, it will be seen, I have also cited some such cases.

Dr. RICHARD EAGER, to whom I have referred in Chapter VI, stated in his Report on Head Injuries during the recent war (*Journal of Mental Science*, 1920), that he had only three cases of serious injury to the temporal region. *One* of these suffered from maniacal excitement, as we should expect, according to our theory. *Another* is claimed by him as melancholic; but, in reality, complained only of pain in the head, and got well on "persuasion". The *third* seemed confused, and wandered about aimlessly. There were three other cases of injury in the *posterior* region of the temporal bone (the area connected with "Delusions of Persecution"), and one of these is mentioned as suffering from "an acute hallucinatory state, and was for weeks in a state of acute maniacal excitement".

On the other hand—as I have mentioned in the previous chapter—Dr. Eager reported a case, which for some reason he included under parietal injuries, and described as "moral deficiency", but which, by his own description, must have originated in the temporal lobe. "A soldier was wounded by a shell splinter *just above the pinna of the right ear*, since when he has quite changed in his character. He is now noted as showing mistrust, insubordination, laughing in his officers' faces, on parade, and seeming to have lost all discipline. Formerly "a staunch teetotaller, he has now taken to drink, and seems to have no power to resist the temptation. Since his head injury, he has been reduced to the ranks."

When the tendency to irascibility is innate, there need be no temporal lesion; but injury or disease of the frontal lobes may, owing to the loss of control, give it exaggerated activity. I have not come across a single case of irascibility in which the lesion was limited to the parietal lobe, except in that form of melancholia called "agitated" melancholia; just as

I have failed to find a single case of melancholia in which the disease was limited to the temporal lobes. With the agitation caused by delusions of persecution, I shall deal next.

Delusions of Suspicion in Lesions of the Parieto-Temporal Area

I have shown that the posterior parietal area has some relation to the emotion of fear, and to anxious melancholic states; and that the lower temporal area is related to the emotion of anger, to irascibility, and, in its morbid state, to acute mania. Now, the area between these two regions —more especially the *posterior temporal region* adjoining the parieto-occipital convolutions—seems, not infrequently, to give rise to delusions of suspicion, as may be seen from the large number of cases quoted. Consequently, such delusions may occur as complications in melancholia, as well as in acute mania. The latter two are merely extensions of disease already existing, from the central parietal area, in melancholia; and from the inferior temporal area to the posterior superior temporal region in acute mania.

Morbid suspiciousness, and delusions of persecution, can arise, particularly in young people, from causes other than a limited brain lesion: as an exaggeration of a natural disposition to taciturnity and distrustfulness; the desire to seek solitude; from sensitiveness of character; and a hypochondriacal condition. Such people begin to interpret everything that happens in a bad sense, and as intended to do them harm. They suspect everybody and everything; they see hostility everywhere; they are constantly on their guard; and the most trifling incidents acquire, in their eyes, an extraordinary importance. Sometimes they begin to imagine that everybody is looking at them. All the words they hear they refer to themselves. Gradually they suspect people of spying, and listening at the door; and following them, when going out. Their mistrust makes them exceedingly reserved. For a time they struggle against their delusions, recognising the possibility that they are such; but, gradually, their delusions assume a more systematised form; they then accuse a certain person, or persons, authorities, or societies, of conspiring against them; and for definite reasons—which they can make very plausible. They now think themselves important personages, to be the object of so much hate, conspiracy, or other unpleasant attention, on the part of their fellow-creatures.

At this stage, or even before, actual hallucinations may set in, the principal one being that of hearing. Hallucinations of sight are extremely rare in these cases—the sight centre not being in the temporal lobe; but hallucinations of smell and taste are not uncommon, hence the idea of being poisoned. These hallucinations of hearing are generally of a threatening nature.

It has already been shown that epilepsy frequently involves the temporal lobes. Consequently, on the one hand, the violence and homicidal tendency of many epileptics, and, on the other hand, the hallucinations of hearing, and delusions of persecution. This observation was also made by Parant (*Archives Cliniques de Bordeaux*, 1895).

Examples of Lesions of the Posterior Part of Temporal Lobes Followed by Delusions of Suspicion and Persecution

I. *Examples of Cases of Surgical Treatment, Resulting in Recovery*

Edwin Goodall.	Lancet, 1898. *Ear disease. Violent.*
W. Rhys Williams.	Journal of Mental Science, 1879. *Ear disease.*
Damer Harrison.	Ibidem, 1902.
E. Amberg.	Journal of Nerv. and Ment. Dis., 1906. *Ear disease.*
Henry Maudsley.	Lessons of Materialism, 1879. *Homicidal.*

Chas. Phelps.	Traumatic Injuries of the Brain, 1898.
W. Sohier Bryant.	Annals of Otology, 1905.
J. M. Köppe.	Archiv. f. Ohrenkeilkunde, 1875. *Ear disease.* Operated ten years after accident.
G. Burckhardt.	Allg. Zeitschr. f. Psychiatrie. *Three cases.*
E. Régis.	Annales Médico-Psychologiques, 1882. *Ear disease.* Nine years after accident.
B. Ball.	L'Encéphale, 1882. *Ear disease. Violent.* Nine years after injury.

II. *Examples of Cases of Injury not Surgically Treated*

Thomas Drapes.	Journal of Mental Science, 1904. *Ear disease. Homicidal.*
Conolly Norman.	Ibidem, 1894. *Softening of temp. lobes. Violence.*
John Keay.	Ibidem, 1894. *Homicidal.*
Leonardo Bianchi.	The Mechanism of the Brain. *Softening. Violence.*
J. R. Eskridge.	Journal of Nerv. and Ment. Dis., 1889.
Chas. W. Burr.	Journal of Am. Med. Assoc., 1907. *Word-deaf. Violent.*
Julius Kratter.	Friedreich's Blätter f. ger. Med., 1889. *Ear disease.*
W. Fränkel.	Allg. Zeitschrift f. Psychiatrie, 1869. *Medico-legal case.*
A. Köhler.	Ibidem, 1877. *Softening of temp. lobe. Violent. Medico-legal case.*
Albert Rosenthal.	Centralblatt f. Nervenheilkunde, 1884. *Developed epilepsy.*
Paul Schüller.	Psychosen nach Kopfverl., 1882. *Homicidal.*

W. C. Sullivan, then Medical Officer, Holloway Prison, later one of H.M. Prison Commissioners, wrote (*Lancet*, 1911):

"Case of Dr. R. Cunnyngham Brown, of H.M. Convict

Prison, Parkhurst: "Patient had murdered his wife. While awaiting trial, he complained of visual and auditory hallucinations, and developed a *persecutory delirium*. After a period of remission, the persecutory symptoms recurred, with increasing mental confusion and apathy, and the patient died some 17 months after the crime. At the post-mortem examination, a large *tumour* was found infiltrating the right *temporo-sphenoidal lobe*." Dr. Sullivan continued: "So far as I am aware, this is the only case on record of actual homicide in this disease." But here are:

III. *Other Examples of Tumours in the Posterior Temporal Region Accompanied by Persecutory Delusions*

James Collier.	British Medical Journal, 1920. *Violent.*
R. M. Marshall.	Journal of Mental Science, 1909. *Homicidal.*
F. J. Mann & Strachan.	State Hospitals' Bulletin, 1891. *Homicidal.*
Berthold Pfeifer.	Allg. Zeitschr. f. Psychiatrie, 1910. *Homicidal.* Two cases, Nos. 24 and 33.
A. Hartmann.	Archiv. f. Psychiatrie, 1884. *Homicidal.*
H. Schüle.	Sektionserg. b. Geisteskr., 1874. *Homicidal.*
Henri D. Dagonet.	Annales Médico-Psychologiques, 1882. *Homicidal.*

IV. *Cases of Inflammation of the Posterior Part of the Temporal Lobes*

W. Julius Mickle.	Journal of Mental Science, 1883.
C. Price Tanner.	Brain, 1890. *With word-deafness.*
George H. Savage.	Ibidem, 1878.
W. C. Hood.	Journal of Psychological Medicine, Vol. XI.
G. C. Gablett.	American Journal of Insanity, 1877.
P. Deecke.	Ibidem, 1882.
T. Duncan Greenless.	Ibidem, 1887.
T. C. Shaw.	Archives of Medicine, 1882.
C. K. Mills & Spiller.	Journal of Nerv. and Ment. Dis., 1907.

Edwin W. Day.	Annals of Otology, 1911.
H. Schüle.	Sektionserg. b. Geisteskr., 1874.
F. Jolly.	Archiv. f. Psychiatrie, 1872. *Bullet wound.*
H. Crammer.	Ibidem, Vol. XXI.
W. Fränkel.	Allg. Zeitschr. f. Psychiatrie, 1869.
O. Hebold.	Ibidem, 1894.
R. v. Krafft-Ebing.	Uber d. d. Geh. u. Kpfv. herv. psych. Krankh., 1868.
L. Schlager.	Zeitschr. f. Ges. d. Aerzte z. Wien, Vol. XIII.
Landerer & Lutz.	Christophsbad As. Report, 1878. *Two cases.*
Tomaschewsky & Simonowitsch.	Wjestnik psichiatrii i Nevropatologii, 1888.
Ch. Vallon.	L'Encéphale, 1881.
J. B. M. Parchappe.	Traité de la Folie.
D. B. M. Bourneville.	Archives de Neurologie, 1880.
F. Baizer.	Gazette Médicale de Paris, 1884.

It has been observed, by several authorities, that chronic middle ear disease may produce a psychosis. Whether this connection is dependent on increased intracranial pressure, direct meningeal irritation, reflex nervous conditions, or disturbed cerebral circulation, is not determined. But the fact remains that, in these cases, cure of the ear disease cures the psychosis (see cases quoted), and if pus is formed, and retained, the mental defect is aggravated.

The general suspicion and paranoid tendency of partially deaf persons is well known. Luther ascribed his incessant head-noises to the machinations of the devil.

Dean Swift suffered from middle ear disease, which gave rise to insane suspicion and irritability, and from this may have resulted his cruelty to Stella.

Subcortical and cortical tumours in the neighbourhood of the auditory centre are liable to induce hallucinations of hearing.

Whenever we get unreasonable suspicion or delusions of persecution, we should examine for ear disease, and inquire for hallucinations of hearing. FISHER (*American Journal of Insanity*, 1888) found only two exceptions in 47 cases of mania of persecution that came under his notice. REDLICH and KAUFFMANN found 90 per cent. of paranoia cases among patients suffering from ear trouble. W. S. BRYANT claimed 50 per cent.; but put nearly the whole of the remaining cases under "dementia". BOUCHERON (*Gaz. des Hôpitaux*, 1887) observed mental troubles of suspicion and persecution to accompany ear discharge. So did C. FÜRSTNER.

Again, increased pressure alone seems to suffice to set up delusions; and the moment pus escapes from the ear, the mental trouble disappears.

A. MARIE (*Archives de Neurologie*, 1898) said that patients subject to systematised persecution delirium had mostly auditory hallucinations. LASÈGUE laid special value on this fact, which is rather underrated to-day.

W. T. TIGGES (*Allg. Zeitschrift f. Psychiatrie*, 1888) has shown that, in this form of insanity, the weight of the frontal lobes is least diminished; next come the parietal lobes; and the *temporal lobes suffer the greatest diminution.*

Dr. JAMES COLLIER, at the Royal Society of Medicine, is reported to have said (*British Medical Journal*, 1904):

"*He could only recall four cases, in which operations upon the brain had been followed by insanity.* Three cases were almost identical. They were cases of tumour, of considerable size, situated in the *central* region of one hemisphere. A wide extirpation was performed. The shock of the operation was profound in all, and *mania of a violent type* appeared early on the third day after operation, and persisted till death occurred within a fortnight. There were in none of these cases antecedents of family or of personal insanity, of alcohol, or syphilis. Nor had any sepsis occurred; nor was any obvious cause of death found at autopsy. The fourth case—one of a large and old-standing *tumour of the right occipito-temporal region*—widely decompressed by Mr. Sargent, developed delusions a week after the operation and became *suspicious*, erotic, and dirty. He was eventually placed under certificate; but six months later his mental state recovered, and remained normal till his death, two years afterwards, from haemorrhage into the growth. It seemed that operations upon the brain, and *serious injuries to the brain, did not give rise to insanity much more frequently than did operations and injuries to less vital structures.*"

It will be noticed that Dr. Collier's first three cases were suffering from violent mania and that the seat of lesion, in the centre of the hemisphere, very likely affected the cortex of the temporal lobes; and that the fourth case—that of a tumour in the *occipito-temporal* region, with definite delusions of *suspicion*—corresponds with my localisation of such symptoms. After the hundreds of cases I have given, it must be evident, to any impartial observer, that injuries to the brain do cause mental disorders very frequently; and that they vary according to the locality involved.

Other Hypothetical Localisations

Physicians who do not believe in the localisation of mental functions in the brain are not likely to put cases on record either for or against the theory. Therefore, all the cases I have quoted, and am about to quote, are purely accidental cases; that is to say, recorded without any afterthought. This makes it all the more surprising that so many cases may be found in medical literature giving the identical localisations; at all events, as regards the emotions of fear and anger, But, when we inquire into the possibility of localising such primary instincts as the *food instinct* and the *hoarding instinct*, it would require more careful search than I have undertaken. Still, the few cases I am going to quote may help those who wish to investigate the matter further.

N. C. Paulesco (*Arch. Intern. de Physiologie*, 1922) claimed to have found the *food instinct* to be located in the inferior part of the frontal lobe (adjoining Ferrier's gustatory centre at the tip of the temporal lobe), by irritation and destruction of this area in animals. But I shall cite cases of *abnormal hunger and thirst* (voracious appetite for food or drink) consequent upon lesions of the *anterior end of the temporal lobe.*

Hermann Nothnagel (*Virchow's Archiv*, 1887) wrote: "A man, age 33, in consequence of a kick by a horse, fell, and came down with his right ear against a piece of wood. He was stunned, and unable to rise. Half an hour later he felt great thirst. He was still suffering from thirst a fortnight after the accident, when he left the hospital at his own request. Within three hours of the accident, he drank five pints of fluid; next day, twenty-one and a half pints; the day after, thirty-two and a half pints; the seventh day, twenty-eight pints; on the eleventh day, thirty and a half pints. A few days later, when he left the hospital, his average had fallen to nine pints. There was no dryness of the mouth or throat, and the skin acted freely. The urine was clear, acid, free from sugar and albumen."

J. B. F. Descuret (*Archives Générales de Medicine*, 1860): A man fell from a high scaffold, and was removed to hospital. He had a contused wound of the temple, and haemorrhage from the left ear. "When he recovered consciousness after five days, he was agitated, and constantly asked for food and drink. He drank daily from seven to twelve pints. He would call at the top of his voice for food and drink, and on one occasion he drank twenty-four and a half pints in one day. After some weeks his thirst slowly abated, and he left the hospital in good health, eight weeks after admission."

OTHER EXAMPLES OF LESIONS OF THE ANTERIOR TIP OF THE TEMPORAL LOBES, FOLLOWED BY VORACIOUS APPETITE, HUNGER, AND THIRST

Percy & Laurent.	Dictionnaire des Sciences Médicales. Article *Homophage.*
Percy & Laurent.	Annales de la Méd. Phys., 1832.
Putawski.	Lancet, 1890. *Injury.*
Thomas Smith.	Ibidem, 1879.
Thomas Smith.	Clinical Society's Transactions, 1897.
W. H. Bennett.	Ibidem, 1897. *Injury.*
Stephen Paget.	Ibidem, 1897.
W. S. Coleman.	Ibidem, 1897.
Kingston Fowler.	Ibidem, 1897.
Jas. Crichton-Browne.	British Medical Journal, 1873. *Tumour.*
E. V. Levinge.	Ibidem, 1878. *Tumour.*
F. C. Wallis.	Ibidem, 1897.
E. F. Brodie.	American Practitioner, 1880. *Bullet wound.*
Monro.	Morbid Anatomy of the Stomach.
C. P. Johnson.	American Journal of Insanity, 1853.
Mortimer.	Philosophical Transactions, Vol. XIII.
Kenneth MacLeod.	Journal of Mental Science, 1861.
S. W. D. Williams.	Ibidem, 1869.
W. J. Mickle.	Ibidem, 1885.
B. B. Fox.	Ibidem, 1891.
Baudin.	Revue Générale de Médecine, 1860. *Injury.*
Bleynie.	Dissertation sur l'Inflammation du Cerveau.
F. Lallemand.	Recherches Anat.-Path. sur l'Encéphale, 1830.
J. P. Falret.	Bull. d. l. Soc. Anat. de Paris, Vol. XII.
Wernicke & Friedländer.	Fortschritte der Medizin, 1883.
N. Friedreich.	On Intracranial Tumours, 1853. *Tumour.*
Rider.	Cited by Schuster: "Tumours". *Tumour.*
Rudolf Ahlers.	Über Schädelschüsse, 1918. Case 71. *Bullet wound.*
H. Schüle.	Sectionserg. b. Geisteskranken, 1874.

PLATE XIX

THREE CRIMINAL HEADS

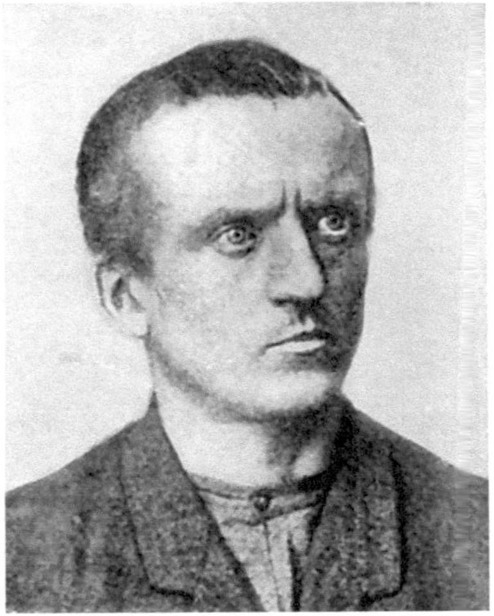

Burglar

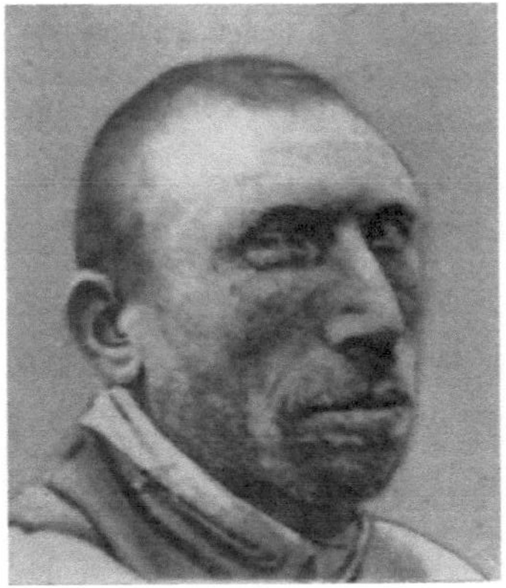

Irish Pig Driver, committed for rape and manslaughter

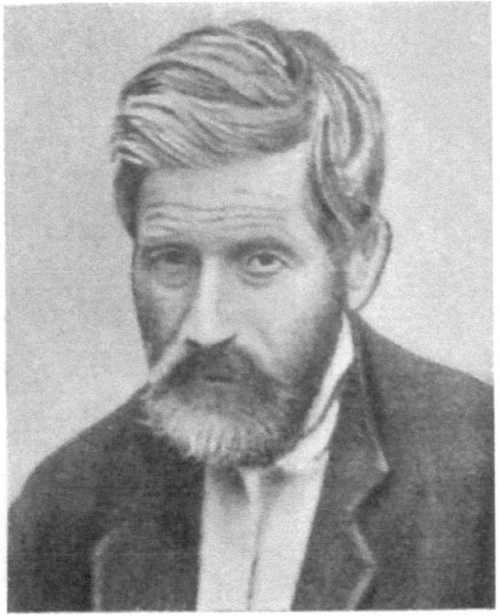

Feeble-minded tramp, committed for arson

R. v. Krafft-Ebing.	Über d. d. Geh. u. Kopfv. herv. psych. Krankheiten, 1868.
Landerer & Lutz.	Christophsbad Asylum Report, 1878.
G. Spies.	Casuistik d. traumatischen Manie, 1869.
Rosenthal.	Über Magen Neurosen, 1886.
H. Voppel.	Allg. Zeitschr. f. Psychiatrie, Vol. XIV. *Two cases.*

Cases of abnormal action of the *acquisitive* and *hoarding propensity* have been recorded in lesions of the upper anterior part of the temporal lobes; again, only without intention, which makes the few cases all the more valuable for purposes of investigation.

The hoarding instinct in man has become greatly changed through the substitution of money, and can be seen in its primitive form only in those in whom the intellect is undeveloped, i.e. in infants, idiots, and imbeciles; or where the intellect and the moral sense is in temporary abeyance, as in insanity.

The impulse to acquire and hoard, in its morbid form, as kleptomania, is of most frequent occurrence in the weak-minded. Some people steal without reflection, and merely to satisfy their animal instinct. They will purloin whatever takes their fancy. Sometimes they display a considerable amount of ingenuity and low cunning in their methods of procedure. Acts of stealing occur also in general paralysis, when the patients steal under the delusion that everything they see belongs to them. They appropriate all sorts of articles, hoard and conceal them, and immediately afterwards lose all recollection of them.

Examples of Lesions of the Upper Anterior Part of the Temporal Lobe, Followed by Morbid Love of Hoarding and Kleptomania

W. J. Mickle.	Journal of Mental Science, 1885.
Kenneth MacLeod.	Ibidem, 1861. *Two cases.*

Thomas Smith.	Lancet, 1879.
P. Crawford Conran.	Ibidem, 1910.
Warren L. Babcock.	State Hospitals' Bulletin, 1896.
J. Christian.	Archives de Neurologie, 1880.
Clovis Gallopin.	Annales Médico-Psychologiques, 1879.
Zierl.	Friedreich's Blätter f. gerichtliche Medizin, 1882.
Ludwig Meyer.	Archiv. f. Psychiatrie, 1872.
E. Klebs.	Vierteljahrschr. f. prakt. Heilkunde, 1887.
A. Spanbock.	Neurologisches Centralblatt, 1895.
Paul Guder.	Geistesstörungen nach Kopfverletzungen, 1896.
F. L. A. Kelp.	Deutsches Archiv. f. klin. Medizin, 1872.
A. Köhler.	Allg. Zeitschrift f. Psychiatrie, 1877.
H. Kurella.	Ibidem, 1895.
R. v. Krafft-Ebing.	Über d. d. Gehirn u. Kopfverl. herv. psych. Krankh., 1868. *Numerous cases.*

An interesting case of persistent kleptomania was reported by Professor Lombroso, in the *Archivio di Psychiatria*, Torino, 1882.

The man in question fell, when a boy 8 years of age, from a height, on to a stove, and injured his left temple. He lost his left eye through the accident, and the temple bulged for ever afterwards. He grew up a rich citizen, and was renowned for his sordid avarice. When 64 years old, he was accused of theft. He had kept a set of burglary tools, by means of which he robbed, not only his own servants—whom he frequently changed—but the guests whom he invited to his house, and entertained there. Lombroso very correctly declared that the injury when a youth had caused changes in the brain of the patient, which produced these morbid inclinations.

Another interesting case, because cured by surgical operation, is that reported by B. van den Hedges in the *Medical Record* and *Revue Neurologique*, 1905:

A boy, 8 years old, had a brick thrown at his head, which caused a depression of the cranium at the juncture of the frontal and temporal bones. From that moment the boy ceased to comprehend even the smallest things and *became a thief* and violent. Surgical operation restored his intelligence and character.

In the course of my practice, as I have mentioned, I have seen a great many feeble-minded children, whose deficiency I traced to injuries they received at birth; especially by badly applied forceps, as was evident by the scars which were still visible. I called attention to this fact thirty years ago; and since then numerous observers have confirmed my observations, which will be dealt with in the succeeding chapter. Here, I want to draw attention to four cases of persistent theft, traced to the same cause.

WILLIAM BROWNING, *Medical Record*, 1921.

Case 1.—J. T., a boy, 14 years of age, given to persistent pilfering. "His head was injured by the use of instruments at birth. This left a scar, and a depression of bone, in right temporo-frontal region. The depression is most noticeable, 4 cm. above the orbital angle, to within 2 cm. of the middle line."

Case 3.—A young man, aged 20, with scars of bad forceps delivery, began stealing when five years old, and guilty of incessant delinquencies since that time. "Otherwise the sweetest and most lovable disposition."

Case 7.—Another case of constant petty larceny, with scalp wound in fronto-temporal region.

Case 9.—Man, 27 years old. "Head badly compressed at birth. Instrument marks on both sides of the right fronto-temporal region, extending right back to parietal bone. He would take, or appropriate, any valuables of his father, or the family; would spend money recklessly, and run into debt."

CHAPTER VIII

THE RELATION BETWEEN THE INTELLECT AND BRAIN

I have shown the conflicting results of experimental physiology and histological investigations into the functions of the brain, and the neglect of systematic clinical observation of the disorders of the emotions and instincts. I shall now show that a similar conflict of opinion exists, regarding the relation of the primary intellectual processes and abilities to the cerebral cortex.

The evidence of comparative anatomy is entirely overlooked: that we have some parts of the brain in common with animals; and others, the size and development of which is characteristic of the human brain. If we take the lowest animal with a rudimentary brain, and observe its gradual development of the reasoning capacity, there is a part of brain, corresponding to the *frontal lobes* in man, which increases in size, and is relatively largest in the gorilla, chimpanzee, and orang-outang, reaching its highest development in the human being.

In man, the frontal region of the cortex occupies on an average 29 per cent. (or nearly one-third) of the total cortical area; in the gorilla, 16·9 per cent. (about one-sixth); in the gibbon, 11·3 per cent. (about one-ninth); in the dog, 6·8 per cent. (about one-fifteenth); and in the rabbit, 2·2 per cent. (about one-fiftieth).

As the other lobes of the brain, both in man and animal, show no such disproportion, we may draw the inference that *the animal part of the brain should possess functions—relating to the emotional and instinctive life—which man has in common with other mammals, and that the distinctly human part should be related to mental acquisitions—intellectual capacities and higher sentiments—which are found in animals only in rudimentary form.* Indeed, if we thus study the human brain from a comparative anatomy point of view, and simultaneously animals and man from the standpoint of comparative psychology, we shall get more light on the functions of the brain than by the methods hitherto used.

Further, if we study the growth of the brain in the human embryo, we shall find that those parts which are the latest and highest acquisitions grow last; and, just as the reflective and reasoning faculties are the latest to arrive at perfection, so the frontal lobes are the last to develop.

I shall produce a mass of evidence, such as has never before been put together, to prove that the frontal lobes must contain the centres for the higher intellectual processes and abilities. But, before doing so, let us analyse the opinions of recognised authorities.

I. A host of observers consider *the entire brain* to be involved in all intellectual processes; and they oppose all localisation whatsoever. They are still imbued with the metaphysical notion of the unity of the ego. But, do not the bodily organs—the heart, lungs, stomach, kidneys—work simultaneously? Why, therefore, should not the different brain centres, which are also organs for specific functions, work simultaneously in their respective departments? *Consciousness is only a phase of that nervous work.*

If the whole brain subserved the intellectual functions, we should be unable to explain the idiot whose brain is arrested in growth. For, according to this theory, he should be incapable of manifesting any emotional and instinctive tendency; whereas, on the contrary, his emotions and propensities are manifested all the more strongly for lack of the inhibitory control of reason. The primary emotions and propensities obviously, then, are as much related to the brain as is the intellect. We have seen that all the weights and measures taken of the brain, in its entirety, give no index to the intellectual capacity of the individual. On the other hand, it is not to be overlooked that examples of idiocy and imbecility are not rare where the brain is of average size and shape; and this is due to an insufficiency of neuronic elements—either from accident, disease, or hereditary defect.

It is astonishing that there should still be men existing, who pin their faith to the belief that the brain acts as a whole, whatever the mental function—that the same structure acts in anger, fear, aesthetic emotion, love, scientific observation, and metaphysical thought, for instance. Those who hold that belief might as well say that the same aggregate of brain cells is engaged equally in the functions of seeing, hearing, and smelling; but they do not go so far, because they know it is not true.

MUNK (*Funktionen der Grosshirnrinde*, Berlin, 1881) found that, unlike the other investigators, he could excite the frontal lobe by means of the faradic current, and so attributed to the most developed brain area a sensory-motor function, *controlling the nape of the neck and trunk*. He asserted (*Allg. Zeitschrift f. Psychiatrie*, 1884) that dogs, the frontal lobes of which had been extirpated, and which were observed "for years", showed not the slightest disturbance of intelligence; and, at the Meeting of Neurologists and Alienists, held at Baden in 1883, he declared that he found that *the removal of one frontal lobe rendered the animal unable to bend the back sideways, and that the removal of both lobes made it incapable of arching the back upwards*. He therefore concluded that the function of the frontal lobes, which are the highest in structural

PLATE XX

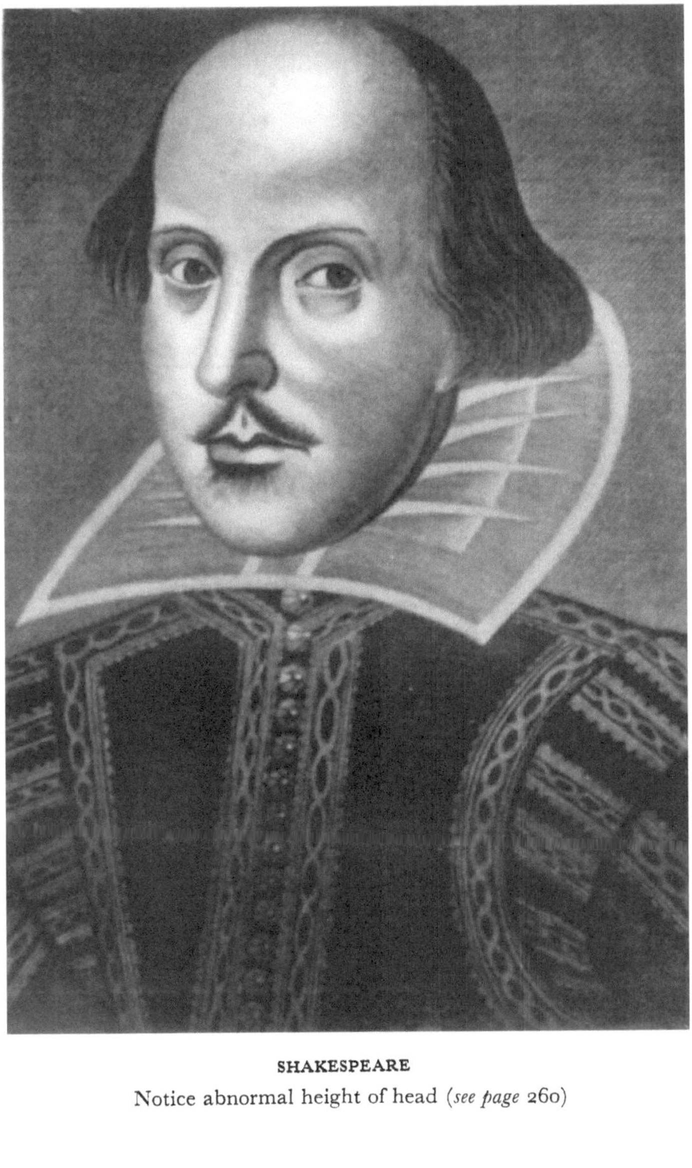

SHAKESPEARE

Notice abnormal height of head (*see page* 260)

PLATE XXI

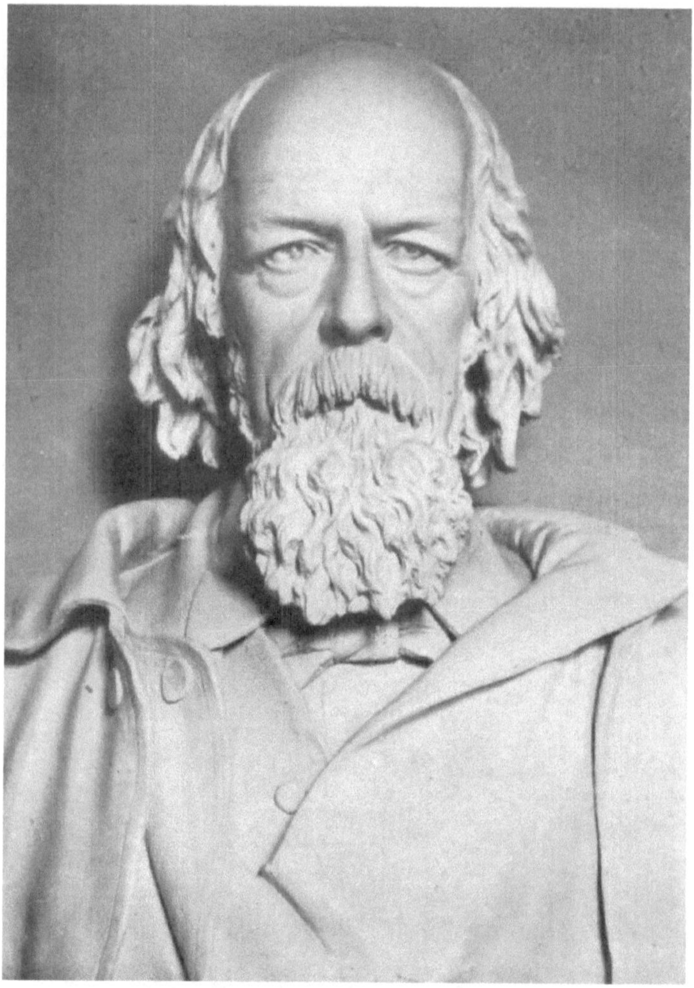

TENNYSON

Notice height of head (*see page* 260)

organisation of all parts of the cortex, was nothing more important than the innervation of the muscles of the back.

HITZIG, on the other hand, found (1884) the frontal lobe could not be excited, and with good reason blamed Munk for having used currents that were too strong. FERRIER, GOLTZ, BECHTEREW, and SHEPHERD, declared that in the monkeys and cats on which they had experimented, they found no disturbance of the muscles of the trunk. The cat would jump and run about, and the monkeys walk and climb, precisely as they did before they underwent the mutilation of the frontal lobes.

THEODOR MEYNERT, following Munk, declared, "Intelligence is localised everywhere in the cerebral cortex, and nowhere in particular".

GOLTZ (*Verrichtungen des Grosshirns*, 1881) also held that "No part of the cortex of the brain can be called the exclusive organ, or centre, of intelligence or feeling; but the psychical functions of sensation, volition, ideation, and thought are connected with all its parts. The quantity of the cerebral substance removed determines the *amount* of the general impairment of the mental powers, instead of the locality from which the removal is made, defining the *quality* of mental impairment." Goltz found only moderate reduction of intelligence, but noticed *loss of inhibition*. His dogs became more excitable, easily angered, restless, and showed a continuous disposition to fight. The facts noticed are similar to the symptoms of mania in man.

Dr. YELLOWLEES (*Journal of Mental Science*, 1898) said they all believed that the brain acted as a whole; and that it was very difficult to differentiate one part from another, in regard to mental and intellectual processes.

HUGHLINGS JACKSON, too, did not believe in localisation of "mental" functions. "For my part", he said, "I think there are not, in the cortex cerebri, any abruptly demarcated centres for any kind of representation"; and he took consciousness and mind to be synonymous, for "if all consciousness is lost, all mind is lost" (*Journal of Mental Science*, 1887).

IVORY, PRINCE, STIEDA also opposed the localisation of the intellect. So did D. J. COFFEY (*Lancet*, 1902).

Most of these observers have not distinguished between intellect and intelligence, Still we must acknowledge that all of them had some ground for their opposition. It is perfectly true that no centre acts singly; we can speak only of centres of highest activity. Any one centre—it has already been explained—on becoming active, may cause the whole brain to vibrate in unison. With reference to the intellectual processes, particularly, we must recognise that, without a motive, there would be no intellectual activity; and that there is, generally, a simultaneous emotion or sentiment, inciting, encouraging, and animating it; and infusing into it the breath of interest.

We must also acknowledge that lesions in other parts of the brain, though they may modify the intelligence, do not destroy it; but we shall show that in lesions of the frontal lobes, one or more primary qualities, and even the entire intellect, may become abolished.

II. A host of other investigators—Carpenter, Bastian, Sergi, Mingazzini, etc.—have located the intellect in the *occipital lobes*.

Goltz (*Über die Verrichtungen des Grosshirns*, 1881) claimed to have found that the disturbances of intelligence which follow removal of the occipital lobes are incomparably graver than those of the frontal lobes.

Crochley Clapham (*Journal of Mental Science*, 1882) declared: "There was no proof that the frontal lobes were the seat of intelligence", for "the occipital lobes occur only in the primates, being absent even in the lowest of the monkeys; whereas the frontal lobes are present in all the mammalia." Dr. Clapham, apparently, was not aware that the occipital lobes are not absent in the lower mammalia, only that they do not cover the cerebellum.

Some of these experts considered the occipital region to be

the intellectual region, because the sight centre is assumed to be in the occipital lobe. As a well-known Edinburgh neurologist wrote: "All knowledge is derived from the senses. The man who can see best, is the man who understands most, and who, therefore, knows what to look for." But the sense of sight is only one of the senses. If, as has been calculated, nine-tenths of all the stimuli which reach the brain from the outside world come from the organs of sight, the blind are dependent on the remaining one-tenth for the scenery of the mental world. But why should the sensory region be just the intellectual region? The feelings and passions can be aroused just the same, and much quicker, as the result of the objective perceptions gained through the medium of the eye. Not only does the sensation of sight arouse emotion, but it differs, according to the emotion or emotions we are already experiencing.

These investigators held to the long exploded metaphysical view that all knowledge is derived from sensation, and that, therefore, the sensory centres, especially those of sight in the occipital lobes, are the centres for the intellectual operations; quite ignoring the fact that man has hereditary tendencies towards certain intellectual capacities, varying for example—as cannot be too often repeated—in memory for words, figures, appreciation of time, memory of dates, facts and events, musical airs, artistic and poetic faculty, etc. Further, they quite ignore the fact that the occipital region preponderates in the lower races and the monkey species, almost in the same proportion as the frontal region preponderates in civilised man (see Elliot Smith and Brodmann); and that the frontal lobes, structurally, are the most perfect. They fail, also, to bear in mind that animals and savages have keener and, in many respects, more perfect senses than civilised man, and should, therefore, if this view were correct, be his superior in knowledge and understanding.

The sensory centres are not the centres for intellectual activity, for knowledge does not depend on sensation alone. What sensation does is to rouse the mechanism of the brain centres for the primordial dispositions to activity, according to their relative development and associative arrangement. The senses are perfected in childhood, long before the structure of the brain is completed. The gradually increasing intelligence displayed throughout infancy and youth is due, to a large extent, to the completion of the cerebral organisation; and talents are sometimes displayed in later years of which there was no suspicion during the process of education. If all knowledge were a knowledge of sensations, the different talents for music, poetry, mathematics, etc., should all be simple modifications of one or more of the five senses. It would lead us to assume that men are born with equal original mental capacity, opportunities and education alone determining the difference of subsequent development. If all our ideas come from the senses, how can we explain Milton, who was blind at an early age; yet what imagination could be stronger, and more brilliant? Laura Bridgman, the blind deaf-and-dumb woman, was remarkably intelligent, and her sister in that misfortune, Helen Keller, has become an accomplished authoress. It is not the perfection of the senses which gives intelligence to the brain, but the perfection of the brain which determines the employment of the senses. External objects act very differently on different men according to their innate mental powers.

III. A number of observers believe the *upper part of the parietal lobes* to be the intellectual area. They fixed upon this region because they believed to have seen *a marked exuberance of cortical growth* in people of undoubted genius. Here we have a revival of the unscientific "bump" method adopted by experts when it fits in with their views.

Sir FRED. MOTT thought that the development of the parietal lobes indicated a high order of intelligence, and is one of the most striking features of difference between the anthropoid brain and the human. (*Archives of Neurology*, 1907.)

LUCIANI located the higher psychic processes in the parietal lobes.

RÜDINGER (*Beiträge zur Anatomie*, 1882), who studied the brains of a number of distinguished men, including Bischoff, Döllinger, Tiedemann, and Liebig, asserted that the higher the mental endowment of an individual the greater the relative extent of the *upper part of the parietal lobe*.

IV. Other observers, however, have fixed upon *the lower part of the parietal lobe* as that in which there is a correlation between a high order of intellect and a relative increase of surface.

According to G. RETZIUS (*Biologische Untersuchungen*, 1898), this was the case in the brains of the astronomer Hugh Gyldens, and the mathematician Sophie Kovalesky. HANSEMANN described a similar condition in the brain of Helmholtz.

GUSZMANN, RUGE, MINGAZZINI (*Lezioni di Anatomica clinica dei centri nervosi*, 1913), BECHTEREW (*Funktionen der Nervencentren*, Jena 1911), and WEINBERG also believed in the parietal lobe being related to a high order of intellect.

Professor D. J. CUNNINGHAM (*British Association Proceedings*, 1901) said, in answer to Rüdinger's assertion that the upper part of the parietal lobe was the intellectual centre: "There was absolutely no foundation for this sweeping assertion. When the evolutionary development of the parietal part of the cerebral cortex was studied, exactly the reverse condition became manifest. It was the *lower* part of the parietal lobe which, in man, both in its early development and in its aftergrowth, exhibited the greatest relative increase. Additional interest was attached to this observation by the fact that, recently, several independent observers had fixed upon this region, as one in which they believed that a marked exuberance of cortical growth might be noted in people of undoubted genius."

V. VICTOR HORSLEY thought that idiocy could be produced by destruction of the *temporal lobes.*

PIERRE MARIE holds the parieto-temporal area to be the intellectual area.

Sir EDWARD SCHAFER seems, also, to have favoured the temporal area more than the frontal. He said ("On the Functions of the Pre-frontal Lobes", *Royal Society Proceedings*):

"The view has been sometimes held that the pre-frontal lobes should be regarded as, especially, the seat of intellectual operations. This idea has been supported, partly by observations of the comparative development of this region, partly by arguments derived from the results of accidents or disease in man, and partly by experiments upon animals.

"I have thought it worth while to repeat these experiments upon the pre-frontal region, adopting a modification of the mode of operating, so as entirely to avoid the shock consequent upon a bilateral removal of a more or less extensive part of the hemispheres. For I have often noticed, in operating upon the brain, that extensive bilateral lesions are apt to be followed by a condition of apathy and apparent idiocy; whether the operations be in the frontal, or in other regions; *more, in fact, in the temporal* than in the frontal region.

"I have, therefore, lately proceeded, not by actually *removing* the portions of brain, but by severing their connection with the rest of the mantle, and with the brain. This can be effected with scarcely any haemorrhage, and with no apparent shock. *The animals have in no instance shown the dullness and apathy previously noticed; but have appeared as bright and intelligent, after recovering from anaesthesia, as before the operation.* These experiments do not, therefore, support the view that the pre-frontal lobes are, especially, the seat of intelligent attention."

VI. Finally, a majority of observers regard the *frontal lobes* to be concerned with the higher intellectual processes. Their opinions will be studied, in detail, in this and the succeeding chapters.

The reader has now his choice of all the parts of the brain where the intellect has been located by eminent authorities. So exact is modern science! Yet, every new result will be hailed as a great discovery, and will decorate our textbooks for a time. It would seem as if each experimenter set out with a preconceived notion, and discovered what he expected to find.

I maintain that the experimenters have failed to discover the location of a single mental quality, owing to the insufficiency of their methods. Because of this failure, a certain number have inconsiderately committed themselves against the localisation of mental functions.

The illustrations in this book prove that the frontal lobes are rudimentary in the different orders of animals, reach their highest development in man, and in different races of mankind and different individuals of the same race are always best developed in those that have the highest intellectual powers.

Numerous authorities will be quoted, who have observed that, when the frontal lobes are destroyed in man, by injury or disease, the processes of judgment and reason are diminished; there is an inability to fix the attention to follow a continuous train of thought, or to conduct intellectual processes; ultimately ending in complete dementia. Moreover, in such men, the struggle between the lower instincts and ethical feelings is diminished, or does not exist any longer; and, instead of a rational man, we see a creature given over to the satisfaction of his lower desires. Such is the case in all forms of lesions of the frontal lobes, and it does not occur in lesions of other parts of the brain.

If we examine the brain of microcephalic idiots, we find that the arrested development is chiefly in the frontal lobes. Indeed, if we compare the frontal lobes of imbeciles with those of men distinguished for their intellectual qualities, we find a great contrast in their size, though the remainder of the hemispheres has attained normal growth. PAUL SOLLIER (*Psychologie de l'Idiot et de l'Imbécile*, Paris, 1891) declared that "Those who are engaged in the education of idiots and imbeciles are aware that the frontal lobes are often defectively developed in those whose power of attention is very feeble". Nevertheless, as I have already said, examples of idiocy and imbecility are not rare where the brain is of average size and shape, caused by an insufficiency of neuronic elements due to accident, disease, or hereditary defect.

Head injury at birth, through bad forceps delivery, is not an uncommon cause of mental deficiency. It may produce haemorrhage, and, subsequently, destroy brain cells, the functions of which, especially those in the frontal region, may never develop; a defect that will be noticed only years later, when demands are made upon the child's intelligence. I have seen a large number of such cases and, in the majority, could discover the scars at the side of the forehead; in the remainder, there was merely a history of prolonged labour or difficult delivery without any external signs. In my various books I have, years ago, drawn attention to this fact; but it is only of late that other observers, apparently from an entirely independent standpoint, have made similar statements.

J. KASANIN (*Journal of Nervous and Mental Disease*, 1929)

PLATE XXII

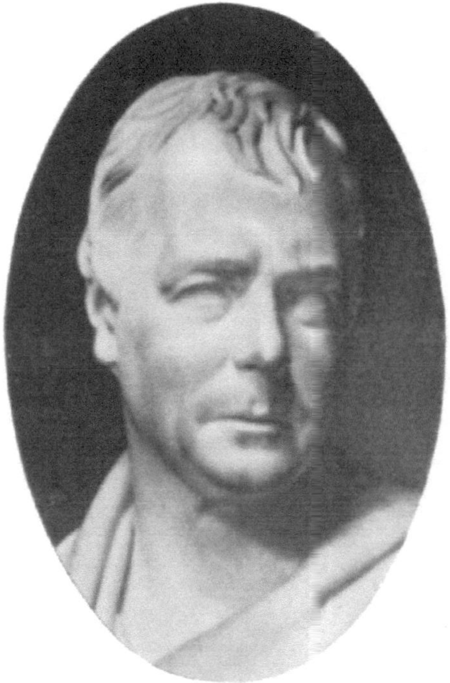
SIR WALTER SCOTT

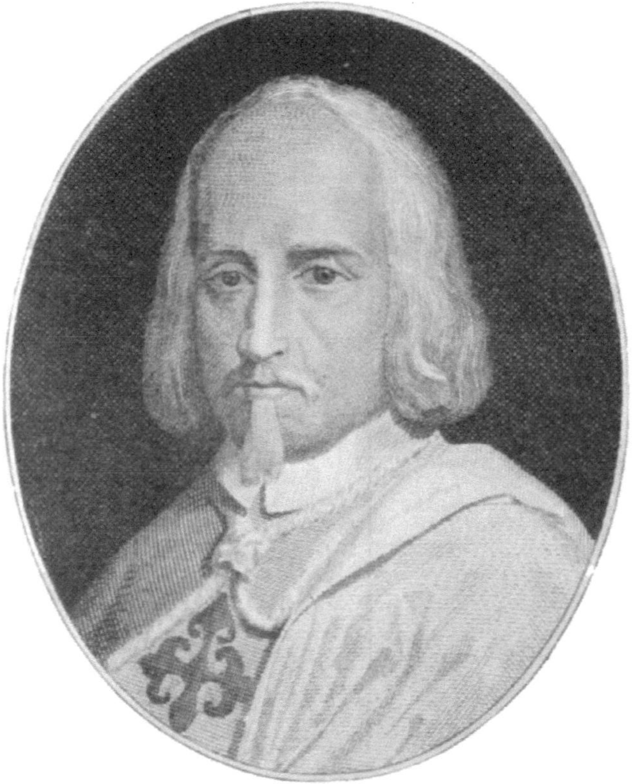
CALDERON DE LA BARCA

Notice height of forehead (*see pages* 101, 260)

PLATE XXIII

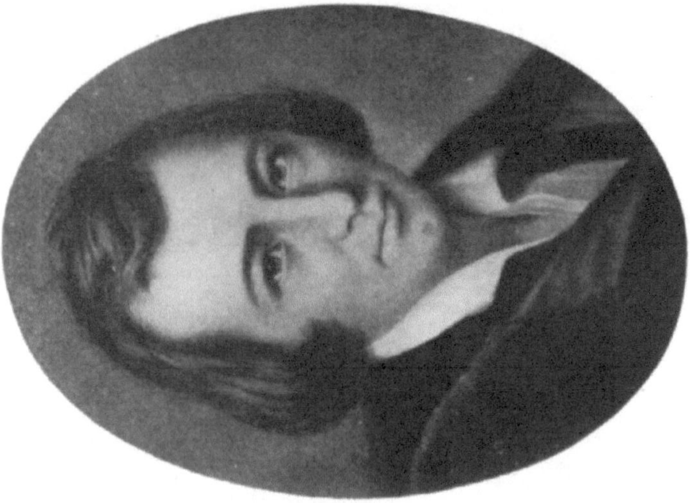

HEINE

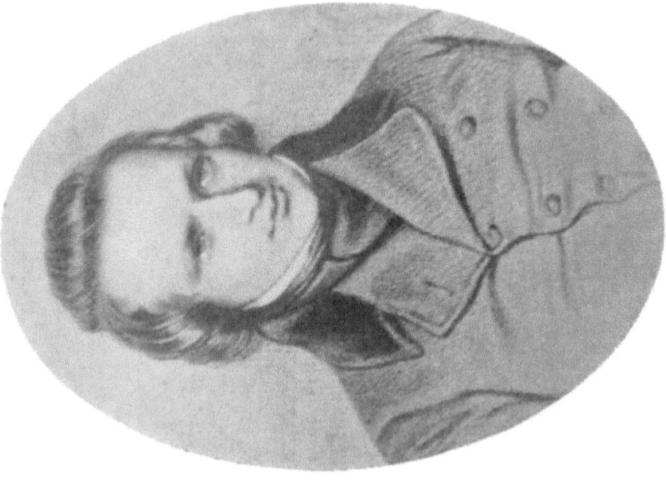

VICTOR HUGO

Plate XXIV

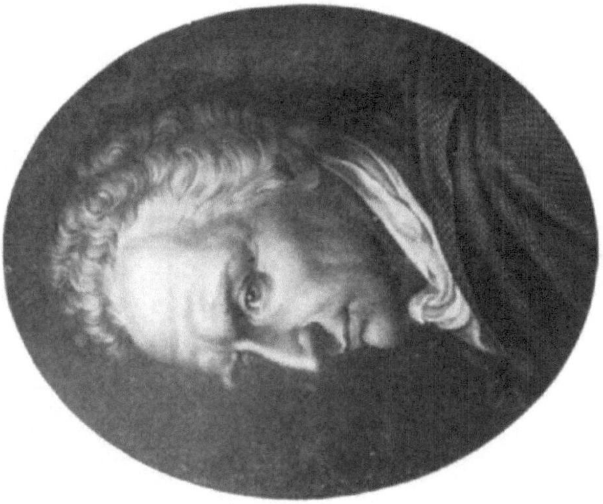

ALFIERI

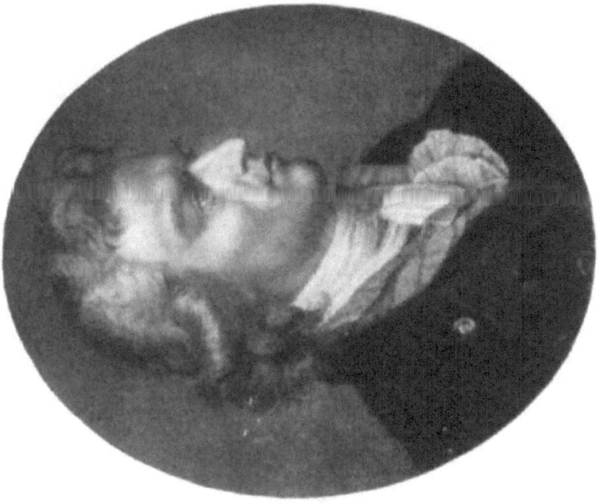

SCHILLER

PLATE XXV

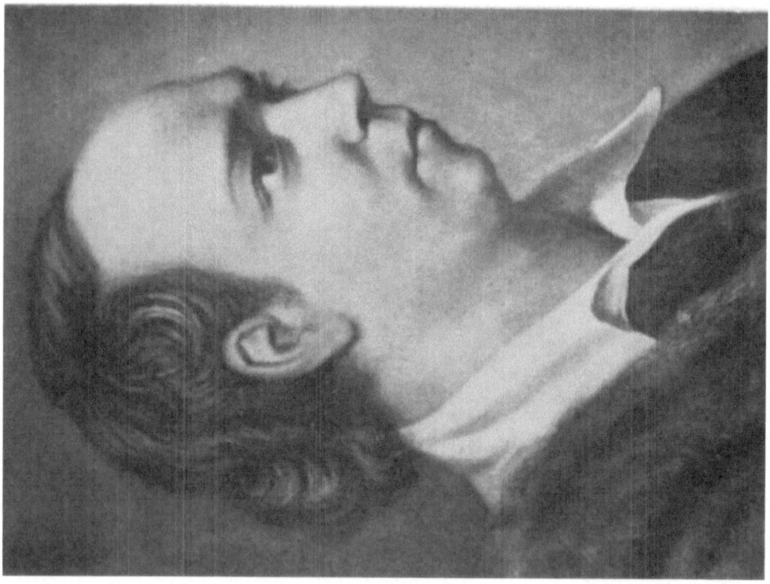

GOLDSMITH

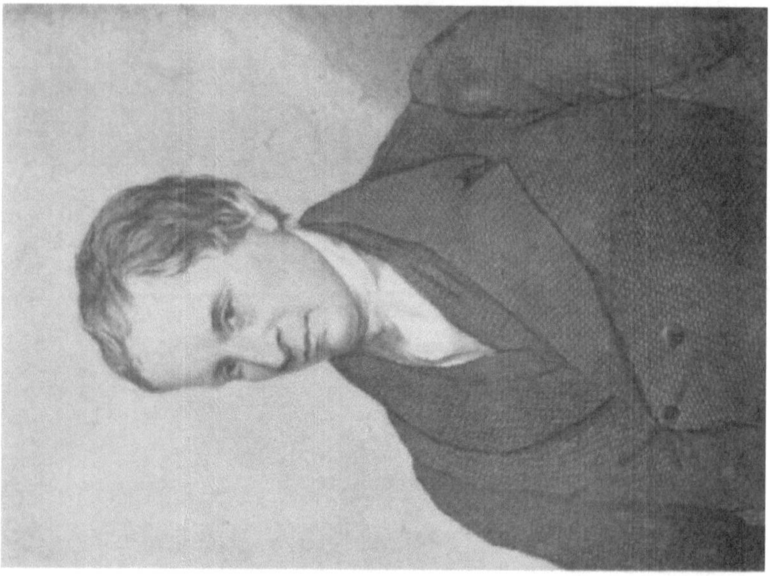

THOMAS HOOD

as the result of a systematic investigation of mentally defective children in a Boston Institution, found that *10 per cent.* of them had received some injury to the brain during childhood or adolescence.

WILLIAM SHARPE (*Diagnosis and Treatment of Brain Injuries*, Philadelphia, 1920), who devotes over 200 pages of his book to the consideration of "Brain Injuries in New-born Babies", said:

"It is surprising how well children under two years of age, and even older, apparently recover following severe cranial injuries; unfortunately, however, it does happen rather frequently that a child entirely recovers only clinically, and if more careful and thorough examinations were made at the time of the injury, and over a period of weeks and even months following the injury, it could be very easily ascertained whether there were intracranial signs present, indicative of future complications—particularly the presence or not of an increased intracranial haemorrhage. In those children in whom the increased intracranial pressure is high, following the injury, although they apparently make an excellent recovery from the acute condition, *yet it is in these children that future complications occur, such as mental retardation and emotional instability*. Their history is so frequently that of being considered normal children, even until the age of puberty, when the cortical nerve cells develop qualitatively as it were, and it is then that the definite signs of impairment appear."

F. C. IRVING (*New England Journal of Medicine*, 1930) stated that "the frequency of intracranial haemorrhage is shown by the fact that out of 182 necropsies, 73 (i.e. 40 per cent.) revealed this condition as the cause of death".

Dr. EARDLEY HOLLAND (*British Medical Journal*, 1923), in his investigations into the causes of death during delivery, observed that in 50 per cent. of the cases death was due to intracranial haemorrhage; and that, *in the majority of cases, the forceps had been used*. Moreover, of the children who are not killed, some suffer from such incapacities as epilepsy, idiocy, imbecility, or paralysis, due to cortical injury. See also Eardley Holland, *Intracranial Birth Injuries* (*British Medical Journal*, 1924); Sir Chas. Ballance, *Intracranial Haemorrhage in the New Born* (*Ibidem*); H. Cushing, *American Journal of Medical Sciences*, October 1905; H. C. Cameron, *Lancet*, 1923.

Animals in which the frontal brain has been destroyed become timid, and easily excited, since they can no longer discriminate. All the emotions and propensities remain intact, but increased in activity, for want of control; but they no longer manifest gratefulness; cannot adapt themselves to new surroundings; neither learn anything new, nor regain what they have forgotten. Experiments on animals thus confirm our view, that the frontal lobes are the centres of perception and reflection, and the centres for the higher sentiments, so far as their rudimentary existence can be demonstrated in the lower creatures; and that they are, in addition, centres of inhibition against the instinctive impulses.

The larger the frontal lobes, the greater the power of inhibition, suspending and postponing the immediate and direct pursuit of an end, a step which lies at the root of all progress, civilisation, and morality. The larger and more perfect the frontal lobes, the more will reasoned adaptation enter into the action of instinctive tendencies; and the greater the self-control.

The frontal lobes contain the association zone for abstract concepts, and complex intellectual processes; and *creative thinking is, certainly, only possible with their highest development.* Their function, also, is to excite the memory cells of any part of the cortex, in the absence of external stimuli, thereby stimulating thought, which may, or may not, result in action.

This is confirmed by Dr. Frederick Tilney, who says in his work *The Master of Destiny*, 1930: "From the facts available it is clear that *human greatness in the main depends upon largeness of brain and extensive frontal development.* The possessors of such brains have been the leaders in the activities of the white man, in every line of his progress, in every detail of his success. They have been the Caucasian thinkers, the idealists, the philosophers, the poets and artists; they have been the white man's pragmatists, his statesmen, and builders of empire. They have also been his spiritual pioneers, the founders of his religion and ethics. To them has been given exceptional power of vision, with equally great capacities for transforming what such vision revealed into benefits for their race."

The brains of Sir William Osler, the great physician, and of Dr. Stanley Hall, the well-known psychologist, revealed as the most striking feature an unusual development of the frontal lobes (H. H. Donaldson). According to Dr. Tilney (quoted above) the brain of the great German historian, Theodor Mommsen, was also particularly distinguished for its frontal development, and so was that of Sir William Bunsen, the scientist and discoverer.

The brain of Laura Bridgman, the remarkable deaf, dumb, and blind woman (whom I must again mention), was studied by Dr. Donaldson, who found the frontal lobes, both in size and richness of convolutions, well developed.

P. Flechsig (*Die Lokalisation der geistigen Vorgänge*, 1896) located in the frontal lobes the anterior association centre of attention, reflection, inhibition. It is concerned with abstract concepts, and other complex intellectual processes. He observed the following changes taking place in lesions of the frontal lobes: (1) active apperception ceases; (2) logical reasoning becomes defective;

(3) loss of ethical and aesthetical judgment; (4) exaltation; (5) loss of self-control.

RICHET, DE BAYER, DURET, GRASSET, P. W. MACDONALD, and many others, expressed similar opinions as to the functions of the pre-frontal lobes.

CHAS. W. BURR, Professor of Mental Diseases, University of Pennsylvania, admitted that the frontal lobes were for intellectual functions (*Philadelphia Medical Journal*, 1903).

Sir CHARLES SHERRINGTON (*British Medical Journal*, 1922) said: "The cortex of the fore-brain was the main seat of the mind."

I shall show—on the strength of a large number of clinical cases, by independent observers—that *over-stimulation of the frontal lobes*, by hyperaemia, leads to rapidity of ideas, a joyful disposition, and, in its trend, extreme hopefulness, feeling of well-being, mental exaltation, delusions of grandeur, and ambitious delirium (a false belief of possession of honours, fabulous property, and extraordinary mental capacities). *This cheerful, hopeful, exalted disposition, is in extraordinary contrast to lesions in any other part of the brain.* In addition, there is sometimes a witty tendency, mistimed humour, and whimsical conduct. Over-stimulation of the frontal lobes leads, also, to loss of self-control, i.e. loss of inhibition over emotions and instincts; and, through the loss of inhibition, the patient seeks immediate gratification of his desires. He is, therefore, morally degenerating.

When the stimulation amounts to congestion, paralysing the frontal brain cells, or destroying them, there will be slowness of perception, and absence of thought from within; responses and actions being elicited only to excitations from without. Further, we shall find forgetfulness of facts and events, loss of logical reasoning, and, finally, dullness and apathy; or else chronic dementia. The higher sentiments get lost, notably the aesthetic; therefore lack of cleanliness is often one of the symptoms.

The commoner symptoms presented by patients suffering from dementia are: General dullness and apathy, a loss of initiative, and an indifference to their surroundings; a marked degree of stereotypism of all the mental processes, and an inability to learn new acquirements; a mechanical method of performing known acquirements; a general stupidity, and inability to understand when an attempt is made at correction of any kind; a tendency to revert to the accustomed modes of speech and action; and, finally, a marked tendency to the repetition of accustomed actions, which often shows that these have been performed in the entire absence of intelligent volition.

This description, in certain respects, resembles that given by numerous experimental physiologists, following the removal of the cerebral hemispheres from certain lower vertebrates, and the frontal lobes from certain higher animals.

HITZIG (*Untersuchungen über das Gehirn*, 1874) assigned abstract thought to the frontal lobes. He pointed, very rightly, to their increasing development in the mammalian scale; the abundance of medullated fibres at the anterior poles of the brain, and the ruin which *progressive paralysis*—that implacable destroyer of the intellect produces, pre-eminently, in the cortex of this region. He said also "It is true that the intelligence exists in all parts of the cortex, or rather in all parts of the brain; but I hold that abstract thought needs a separate organ, and seek for it in the frontal lobes". Hitzig claimed to have observed that *dogs, deprived of the frontal area, forgot all they had learned, and could not learn anything new.*

FERRIER observed (*The Functions of the Brain*, 1876) that "after removal or destruction by the cautery of the antero-frontal lobes, the animals *retained their appetites and instincts, and were capable of exhibiting emotional feeling. They have lost, however, the faculty of attention and intelligent observation.*" He located the centres of reflection and attention in the frontal lobes. He explained: "When the animals have their pre-frontal lobes diseased or entirely removed, they are capable of exhibiting emotional feeling. The sensory faculties, sight, hearing, touch, taste, and smell, remain unimpaired. The powers of voluntary motion are retained in their integrity; and there is little to indicate the presence of such an extensive lesion; and, yet, notwithstanding this apparent absence of physiological symptoms, I could perceive a very decided alteration in the animals' character and behaviour; though it is difficult to state in precise terms the nature of the change. The animals operated on were selected on account of their intelligent character. After the operation, though they might seem to one who had not compared their present with their past fairly up to the average of monkey intelligence, they had undergone a considerable psychological alteration. Instead of, as before, being actively interested in their surroundings, and curiously prying into all that came within the field of their observation, they remained apathetic or dull, or dozed off to sleep, responding only to sensations or impressions of the moment, or varying their listlessness with restless or purposeless wanderings to and fro. While not actually deprived of intelligence, they had lost to all appearance the faculty of attention and intelligent observation."

He also held (*West Riding Lunatic Asylum Medical Reports*, 1874) that "Lesion of the frontal convolutions is, of itself, sufficient to account for a state of dementia. Experimentally, I have found that destruction of the frontal regions of the brain of the monkey induces a condition resembling dementia."

Hitzig's and Ferrier's localisation of the intellect possesses a special interest, owing to the fact that it contains a negation, implied if not expressed, which is more important than the affirmation. Whilst they assign an intellectual function to the pre-frontal lobes, they deny it to the other regions of the cortex.

Lashley (*Psychological Bulletin*, 1928) observed that "no marked *emotional* changes followed the destruction of the frontal region in either cats or monkeys". This is another indirect proof of the functions of the frontal lobes.

BIANCHI (*Brain*, 1895) found, after destruction of the frontal lobes in dogs and monkeys, suppression of curiosity and of the attitudes of observation so common in monkeys; hence a certain degree of indifference to all that occurred or existed in their surroundings; lack of inhibition, consequently greater emotivity. especially a strange fear induced by noises, or by the sight of other animals, such as a dog, the presence of which prior to the operation did not at all disturb the monkey. There was also difficulty in restoring a state of calm (result of decadence of the power of criticism and of the perceptive capacity); defect of reflection, judgment, and memory, and an incapacity for new adaptations. In his own words: "The associative power is greatly reduced. The controlling power of practical experience and acquisitions, such as a normal monkey exhibits in the varied situations of its existence, especially in captivity, which offers opportunity for new adaptations, is absent or withdrawn from the mutilated monkey. Judgment is poor and immediate, often erroneous, owing to the absence of elements of contrast. . . . What is more important is the fact that there is a complete absence of any initiative in those animals upon which the operation has been successfully accomplished. . . . The fundamental emotions are preserved after removal of the frontal lobes, whereas the higher sentiments, so far as these are represented in outline in the monkey, are either absent or profoundly disturbed, corresponding with what is observed to follow severe injury of the frontal lobes in man. . . . In all cases the conduct is seen to be incoherent. This incoherence is due to defect of imagination and of memory, to incapacity to represent and sustain an objective in the focal point of consciousness."

G. ANTON (*Bau u. Leistungen des menschl. Stirnhirns*, 1901) agreed with Bianchi; and COLELLA, too, considered, as a result of his experiments, that the pre-frontal lobes are the seat of the highest psychical functions. "Injury to one frontal lobe has, as a consequence, that the intellectual functions can be carried on only with greater exertion. The memory and judgment are weakened, and continued attention is rendered difficult. If the disease extends to the other frontal lobe as well, then we have sudden and hopeless dementia."

S. J. Franz (*Archives of Psychology*, 1907), after training monkeys and cats, destroyed their frontal lobes, when he found that all freshly acquired habits and knowledge were lost; but, *if any other part of the brain was destroyed, they were not lost.* "This loss cannot be ascribed to shock, loss of blood, or the anaesthetic, for in the destruction of the other parts they are just the same." If one lobe alone was destroyed, the intellectual associations and actions were not lost, but retarded. The emotions and passions were manifested the same as before.

Lussana extirpated the first and second frontal convolutions and the orbital lobes of dogs, and observed that *such animals no longer recognised their master, nor the street or house they lived in. Destruction of any other area of the brain still preserved these memories.* This observation will be shown to be confirmed by a large number of cases of lesions of these parts in man.

Ivory Shepherd (*On the Functions of the Cerebrum*, 1907) found that after mutilation of the frontal lobes, the monkeys lost the faculties they had acquired as the result of education.

G. de Moutier (*L'Encéphale*, 1929), as a result of his experimental and anatomo-clinical observations, came to the conclusion that "the ablation of the pre-frontal lobes in the higher mammals leads to the loss of educability, failure to utilize experience, and incapacity for adaptation to a novel situation—in a word, to a deficiency in mnemonic acquisition".

On the other hand, G. F. Jacobson (*Psychological Bulletin*, 1928) had experimented on the brains of rats, and had found that "The experiments go far toward establishing the complete functional interchangeability of all parts of the cerebral cortex." He had destroyed the frontal region completely, and had observed that *his rats could still respond to psychological mental tests, such as the "maze puzzle"*. If so, then those men or women who cannot solve the maze puzzle may be said to have brains inferior to rats.

The following are a few of the neurologists who have confirmed the observation that lesions of the frontal lobes frequently give rise to serious intellectual disturbances.

CHARLES K. MILLS, late Professor of Neurology in the University of Pennsylvania, said: "The region of the brain in which focal lesions have produced persistent psychic symptoms has been the pre-frontal lobe. If these lesions are both extensive and deep-seated, disorders of memory, will, attention, comparison, and judgment may be present." And again: "Lesions of the pre-frontal lobe, although this is one of the so-called latent districts of the brain, have, in a large percentage of the carefully studied cases, shown distinctive manifestations. The symptoms are largely psychical; and, unfortunately, the physician is not usually well trained to study such phenomena. Mental disturbances of a peculiar character occur, such as mental slowness and uncertainty, want of attention and control, and impairment of judgment and reason; closely studied, the inhibitory influence of the brain, both upon psychical and physical action, is found to be diminished" (*Centres of the Cerebral Cortex in Man*, 1904).

ERICH FEUCHTWANGER (*Die Funktionen den Stirnhirns*, Berlin, 1922) gave a large number of cases of lesions of the frontal lobes, resulting in slowing of mental processes, loss of initiative, abulia, and apathy.

Mental torpor in cases of frontal tumours was found by BRUNS (*Jahresbericht f. Neurologie u. Psychiatrie*, 1898). Also by BRAMWELL (*Brain*, 1899) and PUTNAM (*Boston Medical Journal*, 1890).

HENRI BARUK (*Les Troubles Mentaux dans les Tumeurs Cérébrales*, Paris, 1926) gives *twelve cases* of frontal tumour, observed by himself, with symptoms identical with those described by me in my book on *The Mental Functions of the Brain*, published in 1901, and given in detail in this and succeeding chapters.

BERTHOLD PFEIFER (*Archiv. f. Psychiatrie*, 1910) gives *thirteen cases* of frontal tumour with identical symptoms.

PIERRE MARIE (*Revue Neurologique*, 1919) gives *twelve cases* of injury to frontal lobes with similar symptoms.

FRANCESCO DURANTE (*British Medical Journal*, 1902) said:

"From the summary exposition which I have given, I believe that I am justified in formulating the conclusion that lesions, especially those determined by neoplasms, of the frontal lobes, are nearly always accompanied by *very grave phenomena of altered intelligence*; which proves that the frontal lobes, and particularly the pre-frontal, must be considered as the seat of the most elevated functions of the mind."

C. v. MONAKOW (*Gehirn Pathologie*, 1905) said: "Lesions, of any extent at all, are never observed to occur in this region without causing *the most serious intellectual defects*."

Curiously, PHELPS, the well-known surgeon, most strongly upheld the view that injuries of the *left* frontal lobe alone gave rise to traumatic insanity, whilst lesions of the right frontal lobe were innocuous. He considered that we are left-brained in the intellectual as in certain other faculties.

The following alienists, neurologists, and histologists confirmed the fact that the frontal lobes are most seriously affected in amentia (idiocy) and dementia.

BOLTON (*Journal of Mental Science*, 1906) wrote: "The pre-frontal region is the region of the highest co-ordinating and associational processes of mind." He found (in opposition to A. W. Campbell) that the pre-frontal region of the brain is of extremely complex structure, and of finer architecture than any other part of the brain. "It is the last region of the cortex cerebri to develop; it possesses the highest associational functions; and is the first to undergo retrogression. The greatest amount of wasting in dementia occurs in the pre-frontal region. In cases of amentia, there is under-development of the pre-frontal region, and a more or less marked simplicity of the convolutional pattern. The high grade ament is a man who is required to do a man's work with a child's brain."

O. and C. VOGT found that "the brain formation of microcephalic idiots does not depend on the arrest of development of the brain equally all over; but chiefly of the frontal lobes".

B. SACHS (*Tätigkeiten des Grosshirns*, 1893) found: "Large

porencephalic defects in other areas are compatible with a tolerably high mental development; whereas a defective development of the frontal lobes leads to complete idiocy, even though the remainder of the hemispheres has attained to normal growth."

MOTT, though he did not hold the frontal lobes to be the intellectual area, yet admitted that they were the seat of early and most pronounced atrophy in *dementia paralytica*.

MEYNERT (*Wiener Medizinische Presse*, 1886) observed that "all forms of dementia, including senile dementia and dementia paralytica, are due to brain atrophy affecting the frontal lobes, whose weight is much reduced, whereas the other lobes are hardly at all involved".

P. SCHUSTER (*Mental Changes Accompanying Brain Tumours*, 1902) stated that melancholia and paranoia are hardly ever observed in lesions of the frontal lobes; but that mania and dementia are.

B. MÜLLER (*Archiv. f. Psychiatrie*, 1921), R. VEIT (*Deutsche Medizinische Wochenschrift*, 1922), Ed. MÜLLER (*Deutsche Zeitschrift f. Nervenheilkunde*, 1902), P. HERTER (*Archiv. f. Psychiatrie*, 1915), and H. RICHTER (*Zeitschrift für die gesammte Neurologie u. Psychiatrie*, 1917) recorded cases of dementia (*Verblödung*), in which post-mortem wasting of the frontal lobes was found.

Dementia in frontal tumours was found by BRUNS (*Hirntumoren*, 1895); WEISS (*Wiener Mediz. Wochenschrift*, 1877); HEBOLD (*Archiv. f. Psychiatrie*, 1885); MARTIN (*Annales Médico-Psychologiques*, 1877); BELLAT (*Ibidem*, 1892); STOCKS (*British Medical Journal*, 1874); GOWERS (*Lancet*, 1879); BRAMWELL (*Brain*, 1899); GIANELLI (*Policlinico*, 1897).

Against the view of the frontal lobes being related to the intellect, we have to place the opinion of Ch. CHATELIN and T. DE MARTEL (*Wounds of Skull and Brain*, 1918). These authors came to the conclusion that "there are no symptoms special to wounds of the frontal lobes". They declared that the theory, so long maintained, "that the frontal lobes are a very important centre of association, and the seat of the highest psychic functions, is a purely theoretical assumption", and "has never received the slightest experimental confirmation". They trusted experimenters more than clinical observers, and acknowledged that they based reliance on Munk's "localisation of the trunk muscles", and Sherrington's "lateral movements of the eyeballs" on stimulation of the frontal lobes, and they ignored the observations of Hitzig, Ferrier, Bianchi, and others who observed the mental changes in animals, the frontal region of which had been destroyed. It is strange to find that there are still some authorities who side with Munk (*Allg. Zeitschrift f. Psychiatrie*, 1884), who, as already quoted, found that the removal of one frontal lobe rendered the animal unable to bend the back sideways, and that the removal of both lobes made it incapable of arching the back upwards. Is it possible that the highly evolved frontal lobes have no more important function than the innervation of the muscles of the back?

The evidence in favour of the purely intellectual processes and ability is so overwhelming that we must presume that those who oppose this theory can never have studied the material on which it is based, that they are unacquainted with the history of previous failures, and have drawn their conclusion from isolated cases after only very superficial psychological examination, or none at all.

Even as to the localisation of the *speech centre* which had been accepted for forty years, there is now considerable doubt; at least, with reference to its subdivisions.

I have shown in my earlier books that the French neurologist, Broca (in 1867) was not the first and real discoverer of the "speech centre" in the brain—in the third left frontal convolution, where it overlaps the island of Reil; but he certainly was the first to succeed in getting the localisation universally accepted. In 1868, the celebrated alienist, Dr. Maudsley, still wrote in the *Lancet*: "The truth is that there is no more a special faculty of speech in the mind than there is a special faculty of dancing, or of writing, or of gesticulating." But, with the discovery of the motor centres, in 1871, all opposition ceased. Broca's discovery was based on the observation of only two cases of loss of speech in apoplectics. The third frontal convolution being in the intellectual zone, it is not surprising that it is now claimed that there is no isolated aphasia or loss of speech, but that the intellect is invariably involved.

In the course of time, other observers located agraphia—the inability to express thought in written language—in the parietal lobe; others located so-called "word-blindness", the inability to recognise words, and consequent alexia, the inability to read, in the same lobes; others located sensory aphasia, the incapability of understanding the significance of words heard, in the temporal lobes, and so forth; until the various elements of speech were widely spread over the brain, and a geometrical scheme of their connections had to be drawn, to explain their working. Looking at such a map, one cannot help wondering how little of the brain is left for all the other mental processes; and the question occurs to one's mind: Of what use is the brain to animals, if the identical parts in man are necessary for the complicated apparatus of speech?

In 1906 the French neurologist, Pierre Marie, denied these subdivisions of speech, declaring that the loss of them indicated "a general intellectual impairment". Déjerine and Collier found that sensory and other aphasias are not cortical, but are, most commonly, due to lesions of the white matter, destroying certain connecting paths. According to Henry Head, who is the greatest authority on this subject in England, "there are no 'centres' for speaking, reading, writing, or other forms of behaviour comprised in the normal use of language" (*Brain*, 1923).

Marie's denial caused considerable confusion, and will explain Morton Prince writing (*Journal of Nervous and Mental Disease*, 1910): "Whatever the outcome of the re-investigation of this question shall prove to be, it is evident that the beautifully diagrammatic concepts of the function of language, with which our textbooks were illustrated, and of the aphasic disturbances of this function, in one or other of its many forms as produced by some particularly localised lesion, have been relegated to the scrap-heap of the phantasies of science."

CHAPTER IX

THE FRONTAL BRAIN AND THE INTELLECTUAL PROCESSES OF PERCEPTION, REMEMBRANCE, AND REASONING

The Relation of the Frontal Lobes to the Powers of Observation and Memory

Animals possess a sense of curiosity and power of observation which in some species is developed to an extraordinary degree. The desire to obtain food induces them to examine everything of novel appearance that comes within their range of observation, irrespective of its utility. This curiosity to observe, especially anything unfamiliar, is common to all animals, and their educability probably depends on the strength of it.

Observation is a voluntary direction of the mind to look at a thing which the eyes have seen. By observation we co-ordinate the various attributes of an object, and ascertain its significance. In other words, observation is a mental process by which intellection is added to sensation, producing objective cognition. Our various representations, the different impressions made by the senses, would not exist for us, without co-ordination or association, i.e. without an element which gives them unity, and makes them an object of understanding. We must distinguish between an act of pure sensation and the mental act of symbolic representation. There is a difference between the act of vision—the mere perception of an object—and an intelligent knowledge thereof, as to its nature and qualities.

The sensation must arouse an idea. *Perception is, then, sensation plus intelligence.* The sensory ideas, whether visual, auditory, tactile, or other, are studied, on entering the domain of consciousness, in all their relations to self and the external world. The visual centre may *see* an object, but the perceptive centre *looks* at an object, and ascertains its significance and attributes: their form, size, weight, colour, order, number, etc. It is not enough, therefore, to ascertain that a patient after injury to his brain can see an object; we must also ascertain whether he can see *all its attributes.*

The part of the brain that sees the object is a different part from the one that recognises it. The centre of sensation is not the centre of perception. Sense deceptions, according to this theory, may be regarded as a disruption in the connecting link between the actual sensory and the co-ordinating centres.

External stimuli, in order to furnish mental elements of judgment, must be perceived with the aid and intervention of the attentive faculty. The perceptions must be arrested in the field of consciousness, and recognised. Attentive recognition is what Wundt called *apperception.* It is easy to understand that recognition can only happen when similar, dissimilar, or analogous images are reawakened, when as James would have said, they are called up into the associative fields; or, as the writer would put it, recalled from their respective fields. The frontal lobes seem to enable us to draw upon the centres of the different senses and their memory cells, in the absence of external stimuli; thus giving rise to thought.

It is evident, however, that to assign the faculty of apperception to the frontal lobes is much the same thing as ascribing to them the capacity for recalling, from the sensory centres, those images conserved therein, and necessary

Plate XXVI

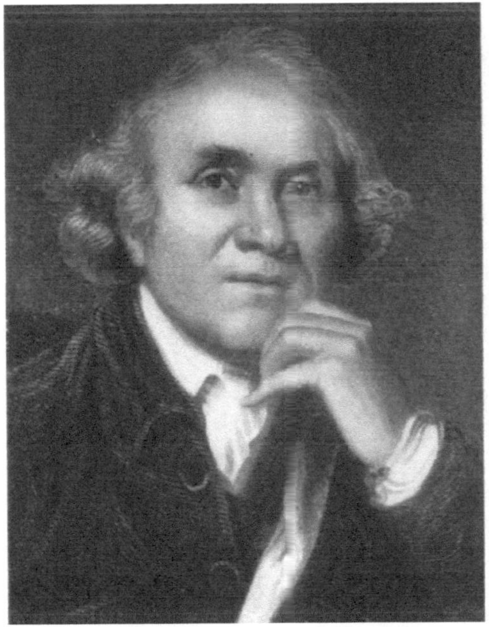

John Hunter, Surgeon
Known for his remarkable powers of observation

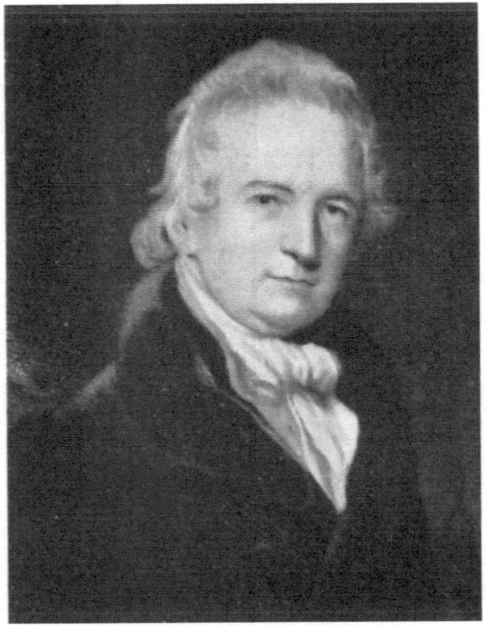

John Abernethy, Physician and Philosopher

(*See pages* 259 *and* 260)

PLATE XXVII

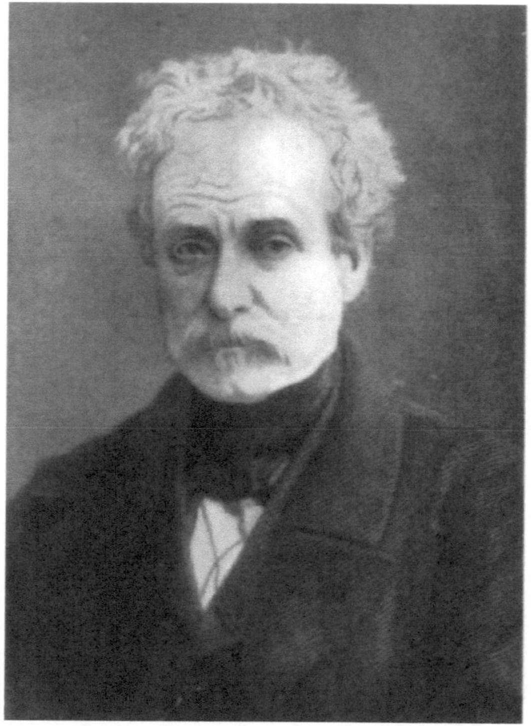

FIELD-MARSHAL LORD CLYDE
Was known to possess a defective memory

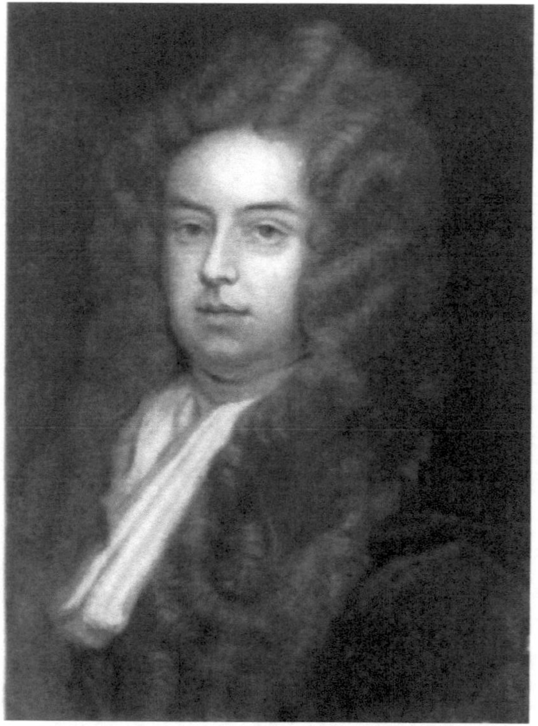

LORD CHANCELLOR SOMERS
Renowned for the excellence of his memory

(*See page* 186)

for recognition; so that in this sense, although Wundt does not say so, the frontal lobe becomes an evocative centre: i.e. a centre regulating the mnemonic function of all the sensory centres.

The majority of physiologists have ignored Wundt's distinction between perception and apperception, and persist in placing these centres in the sensory regions, visual, auditory, etc. Evidence will be produced in this chapter to prove that the centres of perception are related to the lowest parts of the frontal lobes, viz. the inferior parts of the three frontal convolutions, the orbital convolutions, and perhaps the small convolutions within the fissure of Sylvius; and cases will be quoted showing that destruction of these parts causes loss of definite perceptive powers and memories.

Now, an important problem is: *Can mental qualities be localised at all, or only their physical equivalents?* Some physiologists, as we have seen, are willing to admit centres of motion and sensation; but not mental centres. There is something to be said for this view. It is still a problem whether a mental quality, as such, can be localised, or only its physical equivalent—the motor element corresponding to it, and the sensory element which arouses it. But, so long as we do not know what the physical equivalent of a mental quality is, we are justified in speaking of mental centres. It matters not which we locate, so long as we keep both physical and psychical aspects in view. For example, in the process of perception there is, undoubtedly, a muscular element involved; for it has been repeatedly shown that destruction of the frontal lobes, according to the degree of complexity, impairs or paralyses the lateral movements of the head and eyes: movements which are necessary for the accommodation of the eyes, as in the process of attention. When we recall an object, similar movements are performed. When the head and eyes are immobile, there is an expression of uninterest and stupidity, and an absence of active curiosity.

Professor ELLIOT SMITH has shown in his Montgomery Lecture on "Vision and Evolution", in 1923, the correlation of the development of the pre-frontal cortex with the visual area, and has explained that "the sudden expansion of the former (speaking of the brain of monkeys) was due, primarily, to the development of a much wider range of conjugate movements of the eyes, and a further development of the power of convergence . . . so that the animal acquired the ability to appreciate, more fully, the nature of objects on the outside world: their exact position, their form, size, and texture. This stimulated the animal's curiosity to examine and handle things; which not only led to the cultivation of the sense of touch, and the acquisition of higher powers of skilled movement, but also *enabled the animal to train its powers of appreciating form and spatial relations, and to learn by experience the meaning of events which were happening around it.*"

KURT GOLDSTEIN (*Zentralblatt f. d. ges. Neurologie u. Psychiatrie*, Vol. XXX) found—besides lack of fixation of eyes and of keeping the direction—in lesions of the frontal lobes "lack of capacity to discern the essentials of an event". From this psychic disturbance arises inattention, lack of interest and of power of concentration.

The connection between memory and sensory impressions is of the very closest. Indeed, our faculty of *perceptive* sight results from an intimate combination of sensory recollections with sensory impressions. Memory apart, sensation would mean nothing to us. Men with sight only, could see, but would not perceive. Men with hearing only, would hear, but would not understand. There is no sensation that can be appreciated without recollection. There is no sensation which does not call up recollections. It is beyond dispute that the powers of observation are the primary faculties of intelligence; and that they supply the raw material, as it were, for all intellectual exertion. They include *retentiveness* as well, and supply the material for practical knowledge. Without memory, there would be no past, only a perpetual present; therefore, no possibility of comparing past impressions with present ones, or passing judgment upon them. The mind would be the subject of a series of sensations and of nothing more. But, with memory, perception is possible; we recognise the relations between one sensation and another; we can form ideas; we can think and feel.

It is usual to employ the word "memory" in a general sense, to express the property, common to all thinking beings, of preserving and reproducing the impressions they have received; but psychological analysis, and a large number of facts in mental pathology, have demonstrated that memory should not be regarded as a single faculty, having a distinct seat. *Every cell of the brain, and of the body, has its own memory.* If memory were a distinctive power, it would be equally strong for *all* subjects. But, as this is not consistent with fact, we are forced to the conclusion that *there is no general faculty called memory*; but that each faculty has its own power of recalling its peculiar impression. One individual remembers stationary existences; another, moving events; a third recalls, with ease, a train of reasoning; another, musical airs; another, the faces he has seen or the scenes he has surveyed; each, perhaps, weakly remembering something else of the matters now enumerated.

A. A. Friedländer in the *Psychiatr.-Neurologische Wochenschrift*, 1928, gave a case of extraordinary verbal memory, the subject of which was a man who had attended a great festival at which representatives of the State and of the Church made long speeches. This man was asked to make a speech. He did so, and not only repeated the most important sentences of all the previous speeches, verbatim, but even imitated the gestures, intonation, and expression of the speakers. He also repeated, straight through, the Sunday edition of a large newspaper which he had read but once, starting with the editorial, and ending with the last page.

If memory were an independent faculty, it would be equally apt for all impressions, and all subjects. Memory is, really, an attribute, and varies in strength, not only in various persons, but in the same individual. Each special memory of previous observations may become lost, in injury or disease of the frontal lobes; while the others remain intact, and unaffected in the slightest degree. From this we are led to infer that the various memories must possess anatomical independence.

With reference to memory, BIANCHI (op. cit.) found after destruction of the frontal lobes in monkeys, that it became "weak and unreliable, and enormously reduced, not only for recent, but also for old acquisitions. The mutilated monkey does not utilise past experiences; he persists always in repeating the same actions without profiting from the futility of the previous action."

Speaking generally, a man with good perceptive powers is likely to be an observer of men and things: a practical man given to minute inspection, and adapted to study physical phenomena. Combined with the acquiring instinct, he is likely to interest himself in the value of property and goods; and combined with constructive ability, he will be given to mechanical operations, and will interest himself in machinery. A man with good perceptive powers, but small reflective capacity, will be a man of facts rather than ideas, better adapted for carrying out plans than for originating them. He will be a man who looks rather more than he thinks; of quick perception, but possibly little wisdom; a man tending to think nothing is certain and worthy of attention except facts. Good perceptive powers, combined with good reflective powers, make a man not only a close observer of things, but, also, strongly inclined to trace their relations of cause and effect.

A man with small perceptive powers will be deficient in the capacity of observation, and will take little interest in the mere examination of objects; and, if he have superior reflective power, will be more of a philosopher than a scientist, a bookworm rather than an experimenter in the laboratory. That is to say, *he is most likely* to be these things; his tendencies will run in these directions.

Each of the perceptive powers and memories will be dealt with in detail; and we shall show that each of them depends on a definite centre in the frontal lobes. Their loss in the case of brain lesions is rarely inquired into; or, if discovered, is more often located in some distant "sensory" region.

The perception and memory of *form* is commonly accepted as an elementary power. We all vary in it, as, for example, in its application to the remembering of faces. It is said of Cuvier that he was able to recognise a similarity in form in the most extraordinary manner, never forgetting the shape of an object he had once seen. The special memory developed by this faculty is also well illustrated by those artists who are able to draw accurately from memory; thus it is said of Turner, that, having carefully looked at a ship, he was able to go home and draw, from memory, the details of the ship as accurately as if he had been standing in front of it.

The power to observe the *size* of objects is another elementary capacity. Its function is manifestly different from that of the faculty of form; thus, a sixpence and a half-crown are of the same form, but differ in size. Another innate faculty is the power of appreciating *resistance*; or sense of weight. The perception of position or *locality*, giving the memory for places—a natural instinctive knowledge of one's situation—varies greatly in different people, and appears to be more developed in savages and animals than in persons belonging to civilised communities.

The ability to deal with *numbers*, being a natural power, can, of course, like any other, be improved by exercise and practice, but, nevertheless, no amount of practice will produce it where nature has not bestowed it. This numerical faculty depends, also, on no sense in particular. It is a natural gift, and as with other gifts, when there is great ability in regard to it, there is generally also a great love for it.

Another elementary power is that of perceiving periods of *time*, forming what might be termed a natural "chronometer" sense in the individual. This power, likewise, depends on no sense in particular. "Time" memory may be seen in those persons who are able to remember the chronological order of events easily.

The perception of time is essential to musicians; but it does not make a musician. Several other qualities are required. A person with a small development of *tone-perception* thinks music a "noise", and takes no pleasure in it, not being able to distinguish one tune from another.

On the development of the perceptive centres depend, also, in part, the talents of drawing, painting, sculpture, mechanics, etc.; and from the desire to know objects in the relation to their separate existence, our inclination for the study of science arose. Our perceptions and memories may be divided, further, into those of mere existence—stationary objects—and those for moving objects, or objects in time, i.e. for *facts and events.*

E. Niessl v. Mayendorf admits loss of perception accompanying anterior cortical lesions (*Zeitschrift f. d. ges. Neurologie*, 1919).

The ability to recognise the form of an object as well as its nature—the stereognostic sense—may be lost independently. This was recognised by Mills, Hoppe, and Weisenburg, but they located it in the superior part of the parietal lobe; whereas the cases quoted in the succeeding pages show it to be in the orbital convolutions. The independence of the stereognostic sense —without giving any locality—was also recognised by Robert Sommer (*Zeitschrift f. Physiologie der Sinnesorgane*, Vol. II), Bergmann (*Allg. Zeitschrift f. Psychiatrie*, Vol. VI), and Hebold (*Archiv. f. Psychiatrie*, 1885) on the basis of definite cases.

The localisation of disorientation in space has been confirmed by Pierre Marie and Béhague (*Revue Neurologique*, 1919).

Willbrand observed the loss of appreciation of time. Förster (*Archiv. f. Ophthalmologie*, Vol. XXVI) observed the loss of the memory for places. Groeunow (*Archiv. f. Psychiatrie*, Vol. XXIII) did the same. Similar observations were made by Bjernum, Brill, Cohen, Schnelle, etc.

Monkeys are notoriously curious animals; but after destruction of the frontal brain they lose interest, allow many things to pass unobserved, and fail to recognise objects with which they have previously been familiar.

Bianchi (*The Mechanism of the Brain and the Functions of the Frontal Lobes*, 1922) gave an excellent account of the changes in perception following upon such an experiment. One of the results, he says, is "Defect of the perceptive power, consisting in an incomplete perception of the objects of the external world; a perception which is lacking in certain of the specific and differential features, and accordingly gives rise to defective recognition of objects already known, and of new objects having relations of similarity, analogy, etc., with these. So it happens that some objects are mistaken for others that resemble them only in colour or in form. There is, also, a notable defect in the perceptive power, in the sense that, whilst intact, animals let nothing escape them, and are constantly poking about, and taking stock of anything that exists in any particular environment; mutilated monkeys, on the other hand, allow a number of things and situations to pass unobserved."

Goltz found that dogs, deprived of the pre-frontal region of the brain, acted differently from normal animals. Very remarkable is the following experiment which he made. "If a bone is thrown to the animal at some distance, it runs to it with great alacrity, but does not have the sense to stop at the right moment and sink its head; so that it runs beyond the mark, as if it had lost the *sense of distance*. Instead, however, of turning round and looking for the bone in a methodical way, the animal appears to forget what it was after, and runs on regardlessly until the bone is lifted and the animal's attention again attracted to it."

We have seen that, in idiocy, the arrested development is chiefly in the frontal lobes. Now, sometimes, idiot children have talents in special directions, which are all the more remarkable, because of their lack of sense in every other direction. We can only explain such natural gifts by assuming that they are dependent on special centres in the brain, which are rich in neurons, as compared with the remainder of the cortex. It is not uncommon to find, in idiot institutions, children with an extraordinary talent for remembering dates and past events.

Several children under Dr. Langdon Down's care have possessed this faculty to an exceptional degree. One idiot boy never failed to recall the name and address of every confectioner's shop that he had visited in London—and they had been numerous; and he could as readily tell the date of each visit. Another child could tell the time of arrival of all the children at the institution, and could supply accurate records in relation to it when needed. One boy under Dr. Down's care had a very unusual faculty, namely, the perfect appreciation of past or passing time. He was 17 years of age, and, although not understanding so far as could be gathered the use of a clock-face, could tell the time to a minute at any part of the day, and under any circumstances. Dr. Down tried him on numberless occasions, and he always answered with an amount of precision truly remarkable.

Dr. E. T. Boland brought before the New England Psychological Society, October 11, 1887, an idiot-savant, a boy named George, 16 years old, whose strong point was that he could answer questions as to calendar dates in his past life, and for a year or two in the future. He had never learned to read—sight being too defective, even had his capacity permitted. He was an imbecile in every respect.

Dr. Shuttleworth had in his institution a remarkable case of a young man with a history of congenital imbecility who was able, without much mental effort, to give the day of the week corresponding to the day of the month for several years past, and for several years to come. His ready answers were very surprising to strangers.

J. Pereira Gray (*British Medical Journal*, 1919): "James C. is a native of Devonport, is 60 years old, and a certified imbecile. He has been in a Poor Law Institution practically all his life. He makes use of very few words, and has a tendency to repeat the same phrases over and over again. Yet this man, if given the number of any psalm taken at random, can repeat the psalm correctly. He can do the same with any hymn. He can give the right lesson for any Sunday in the year. But what I consider a still more remarkable feat is that, if given any date, he will name the day of the week on which that date fell. I have tested his memory on several occasions, and his answers were invariably correct."

Dr. R. Eager was reported in the *British Medical Journal*, 1926, at a Meeting of the Devon and Exeter Medico-Chirurgical Society, to have shown an imbecile, age 37, who had memorised the titles and numbering of the hymns in the hymn-book from cover to cover, and who was tested by those present.

Examples of the Loss of Special Perceptions and Memories

The Author's Observation of a Case Involving Loss of Form, Size, Weight, and Memory of Dates and Names

E. M. J., a farmer, age 60, received a kick from a horse on his forehead, crushing in the skull at the root of the nose along the level of the eyebrows, the fracture extending upwards to the middle of the forehead, showing afterwards an unsightly depression at the seat of injury. The patient, who remained in a semi-conscious condition for several weeks after the occurrence, made a gradual recovery, but the following symptoms remained. He was able to walk about and look after his farm affairs, but found that he had lost interest. It was noticed that he could not learn and observe things as before; that *he could not remember dates, names, or even recognise faces and forms* as readily as before. He who could formerly guess at distances correctly, could no longer measure them with the eye. Form, size, width, and height seemed changed to him. Formerly a good shot, he could not aim at any object now, a bird in the air appearing a long way off, when, in fact, it would be near, or almost directly over him. Nor could he estimate the weight of cattle, dogs, and horses, at which he was naturally clever before the accident. He spoke rationally, and was perfectly normal in every other capacity and disposition, except that he had an inclination to frequent anger without apparent cause. This was the only loss of control that could be ascertained.

Another Case of the Author's Own Observation, Involving Loss of Sense of Size and Weight

H. B., age 55, a tailor, was during a quarrel hit by a billiard ball over the left eye, fracturing the skull over the supra-orbital foramen. After recovering consciousness, he suffered from agonising attacks of supra-orbital neuralgia, for which he was treated. As regards the mental condition, it was noted that the patient lost control over his feelings, and for a time was considered insane. He recovered, however, completely, and became a normal man, but for the loss of appreciation of size and weight, so that he could no longer cut cloth or fit garments.

Two Other Cases of My Experience, Involving Loss of Memory for Facts and Events

These were male patients who had received injuries to the centre part of the forehead. Both had been married recently, and had forgotten all about it, though they could remember events prior to their marriage. One of them was very positive in his statement that he had never met the lady in question.

Case of Frontal Injury, Loss of Sense of Weight and Sense of Resistance

Thos. Laycock (*Australian Medical Journal*, 1893): A case of fracture of the base of the skull just behind the orbits, there being a fissure about a quarter of an inch in width. The patient, a man age 29, was treated surgically. Much lacerated and contused brain substance was removed. On recovery, patient had lost the conception of the quality and position of foreign bodies, their weight and resistance, as perceived by the sense of touch.

Case of Frontal Injury, with Loss of Memory of Previous Events, of Forms, Objects, and Places (see Illustration).

H. M. Abel and W. S. Colman (*British Medical Journal*, 1895): The patient, G. T., a sober, well-conducted railway fireman, age 36, was brought to the Peterborough Infirmary with the broken ends of an oil-feeder protruding from his right cheek, a little behind the angle of the mouth. It was stated that in stepping from the tender on to the footplate of his engine with the oil-feeder in his hand, he had slipped and fallen forward, the spout of the oil-can being driven forcibly into his face. He was then quite senseless, but in a few minutes partially recovered consciousness. When he was being placed on the stretcher, someone suggested a coat for his head, and he was sensible enough at that time to say that his own coat was on the engine; so that the loss of memory afterwards so conspicuous was not then present. He reached the hospital quite conscious. The metal spout of the oil-can was firmly fixed in the base of his skull, and required firm traction with forceps to relieve it from the grasp of the bone. It passed upwards and towards the middle line, and the concavity of the spout was directed from the middle line; the end of the oil-can entering the skull at the inner corner of the right eye, and reaching up to the middle of the forehead. There was now paralysis of the left side of the face and left arm, while the left leg was little affected. Mental condition: *he could not recognise his wife or his old comrades, but he had, also, difficulty in recognising common objects and their uses.* He did not recognise a fellow-workman who had met with an accident, and was in a bed next to him, for weeks. But, what was the most remarkable was that *the whole of his life for twenty years before the accident was wiped out from his memory.* He asserted he was a farm labourer, which was so prior to his employment on the railway. All the memory of the accident was gone, and has never returned. After he left the hospital, some previous events did return; but, after the lapse of a year, there was still five years of which he could remember nothing. The paralysis had nearly disappeared; but the arm was left weak. There was very little control over his emotions. He laughed or cried at the slightest provocation. His irritability of temper was said to have increased, and he was often hasty in his language, although not violent. The partial return of his memory seems to have been, in part, due to the habit of his "mates" coming in and talking to him of the past,

Plate XXVIII

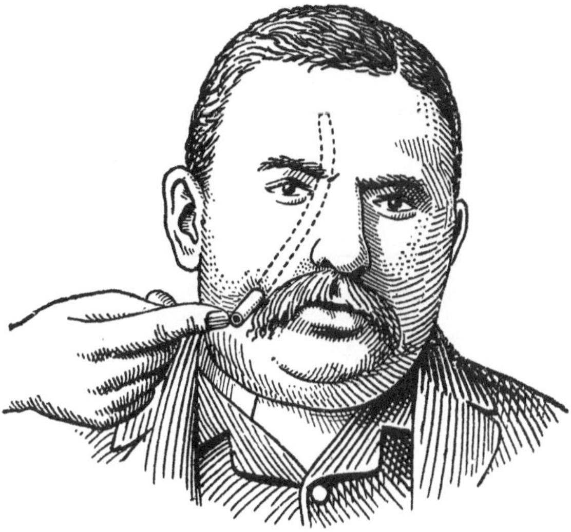

ILLUSTRATION TO CASE OF HEAD INJURY WITH SEVERE LOSS OF MEMORY

(*Page* 196)

Diagram (from a photograph taken a year after the accident) indicating the probable course of the tin spout

and continually reminding him of occurrences which were likely to have made an impression on him. There was still extreme difficulty in retaining in his memory any passing events. If he went out for a walk alone, he was unable to find his way back, and often failed to recognise his own house when he was outside; and there was also frequent failure to recognise common objects and their uses. *There was present, therefore, a condition of imperception.* There was no aphasia at any time, and no difficulty in expressing himself. His reasoning processes were fairly orderly, but as—owing to the blanks in his memory—he often argued from false premises, he arrived at ludicrously incorrect conclusions. For example, he occupied one of the houses built by the railway company for their servants, and as he had no recollection of having worked for them for five or six years, he argued that he had no right to be there, and insisted with unnecessary warmth that his wife should pack up and leave the house before they got into trouble for being there.

Case of Frontal Injury—Loss of Sense of Time, of Locality, and of Objects

J. WENDE (*Allg. Zeitschrift f. Psychiatrie*, 1905): Patient, age 33, fell off a scaffolding, seven feet high, when the right side of his forehead struck an iron screw, and he sustained a wound about four centimetres in length. He was rendered senseless, but soon recovered consciousness. Subsequently, he frequently lost control over his temper, and there was absolute loss of the sense of time, complete failure of self-orientation, and inability to notice things.

Case of Frontal Lesion—Loss of Sense of Time, Memory of Places and of Objects

M. JASTROWITZ (*Deutsche Medizinische Wochenschrift*, 1887): Patient, wife of a major in the army, age 42, had a syphilitic scar three centimetres in length over the glabella, above the root of the nose. Though intellectually quite normal, she could not distinguish either time or locality, and mistook objects. The post-mortem examination revealed inter-meningeal haemorrhage at the anterior root of the superior and middle frontal convolutions.

Case of Frontal Tumour—Euphoria, Loss of Sense of Time, Place, and Number

Gabriel Chèze (*Écho Médical du Nord*, 1910): Marie V., age 42, found wandering in a state of nudity, smiled happily, had optimistic notions, no knowledge of time and place, no idea of simple calculation. Died five days later. A large sarcomatous tumour was lying across the orbital plates of the frontal bone compressing the orbital convolutions, which were partially destroyed.

Case of Frontal Tumour, Accompanied by Disorientation and Loss of Memory and Sense of Time

F. X. Dercum (*Journal of Nervous and Mental Disease*, 1910): I. G. C. I., age 59, book-keeper. "His wife reported that he had been in a 'dreamy' state of mind for some time, and that he seemed to have no idea of time. He often forgets what he is doing. At times he does not seem to know just where he is; sometimes loses himself in his house. His wife states further that he does not seem to notice the change in his condition; that he does not manifest any anxiety about himself. He does not worry, and assumes no responsibility regarding his affairs." Post-mortem, a sarcomatous tumour was found in the right frontal lobe.

Case of Frontal Tumour with Loss of Memory for Facts and Events

Leonida Canali (*Rivista Sperimentali de Freniatria*, 1881): Antoine Ruggeri, age 44, a priest, struck his forehead against a wooden post in his house. Remained unconscious for about half an hour. The injury and subsequent headache was in the region of the right frontal eminence. A year later mental changes followed. He became loquacious, his memory for facts and events got markedly enfeebled, and his ideas disordered. Gradually he also lost control over his character tendencies, becoming haughty, irascible, and intolerant. Eighteen months later he died in a fit. The autopsy revealed a glio-sarcoma involving the middle of the first and second frontal convolutions on each side.

Cases of Frontal Tumour Causing Loss of Memory for Facts and Events were given by

Bruns.	In his book on Tumours of the Brain.
L. Lotte.	British Medical Journal, 1884.
Schultze.	Deutsche Zeitschrift. f. Nervenheilkunde, 1896.
Schuster.	Psychische Störungen bei Hirntumoren, Stuttgart, 1902.
Pierre Marie.	Revue Neurologique, 1919 and 1924. *Reported cases of frontal tumours with "disorientation".*

Examples of Recovery of Memory After Surgical Operation

Cases of Frontal Tumour, with Enfeeblement of Perception and Memory—Surgical Operation—Recovery

Gianelli (*Policlinico*, 1897): Patient manifested slowness of perception and confusion of memory. On removal of the tumour complete recovery.

Case of Frontal Tumour with Loss of Memory—Operation—Recovery

Seydel (*Neurologisches Centralblatt*, 1896): Case of loss of memory, loss of all interest, apathy. Removal of tumour led to complete recovery.

Case of Frontal Tumour with Loss of Memory for Facts and Events—Surgical Operation—Recovery

Francesco Durante, Rome (*British Medical Journal*, 1902): S. D., age 39, suffered from "slow perception", mnemonic confusion for remote facts, and abolition of memory for recent facts.

On operation, large subcortical gumma, involving nearly the whole of the left frontal lobe, was removed. Result: "Complete cure of all the symptoms."

The Frontal Lobes and Reflective Power

The frontal lobes contain the centres for reasoning on the knowledge gained. Consequently, in lesions of the frontal lobes we frequently find that "logical reasoning becomes defective".

The following is a *case of Frontal Tumour followed by Loss of Induction and Deduction, and Recovery after Surgical Operation.*

William Elder and Alexander Miles (*Lancet*, 1902): Patient, a man age 47, had a tumour of the left pre-frontal lobe, *exactly under the frontal eminence,* which was swollen. As regards the affection of his memory, it appeared to be not so much a blotting out of his past impressions as a want of the power of associating memories, of comparing and contrasting them. *Loss of power of forming a judgment about anything* and loss of attention were prominent symptoms of his mental condition. He could not compare or contrast two things or ideas. His individual memories seemed all right. He recognised objects and friends. His emotional condition was another prominent symptom in his case. He lost the sense of modesty and shame. There was evidently loss of inhibition. The skull was trephined, the tumour removed, and the patient's symptoms rapidly disappeared.

E. A. Spitzka, the American Neurologist, who dissected the brains of various celebrities, claimed to have noticed the difference between one who was "more creative, constructive, philosophical, and brilliant in abstract generalisations", and another who was "a far keener observer, quick at seeing analogies, an excellent systematiser, and had a splendid power of memorising and recalling visual impressions" (*Transactions of the American Philosophical Society*, 1907).

Bianchi (op. cit.) said that "destruction of the frontal lobes in monkeys has the effect that the associative power is greatly

Plate XXIX

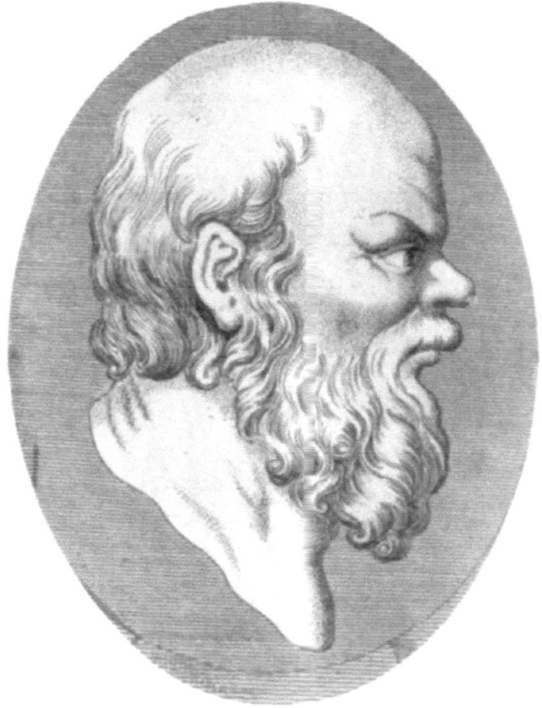

SOCRATES, PHILOSOPHER
Religious

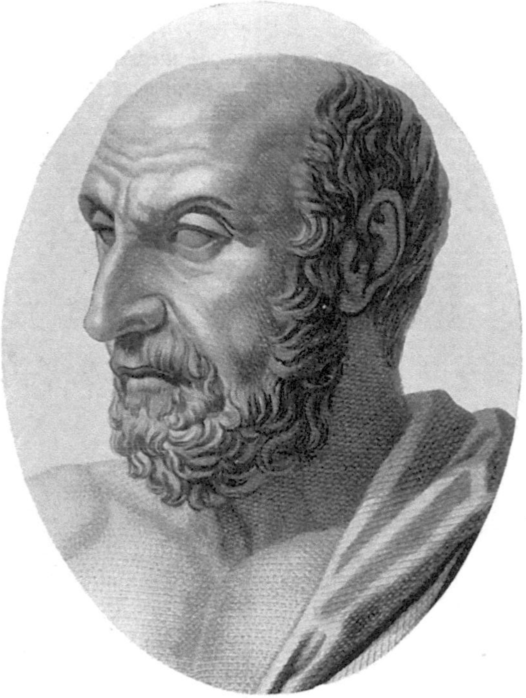

DEMOCRITUS, PHILOSOPHER
Rationalist

(*See page* 260)

PLATE XXX

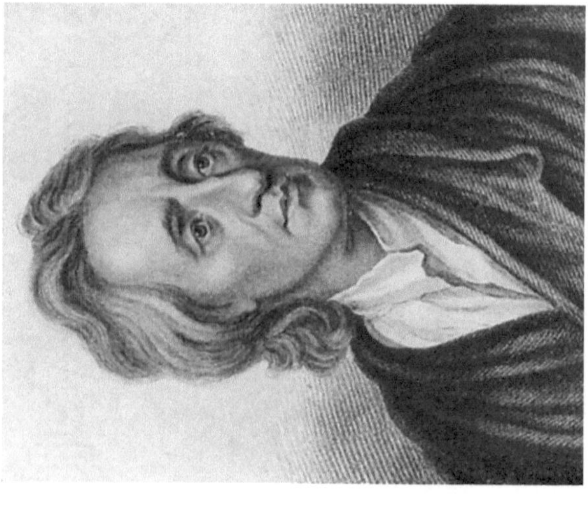

LOCKE, PHILOSOPHER

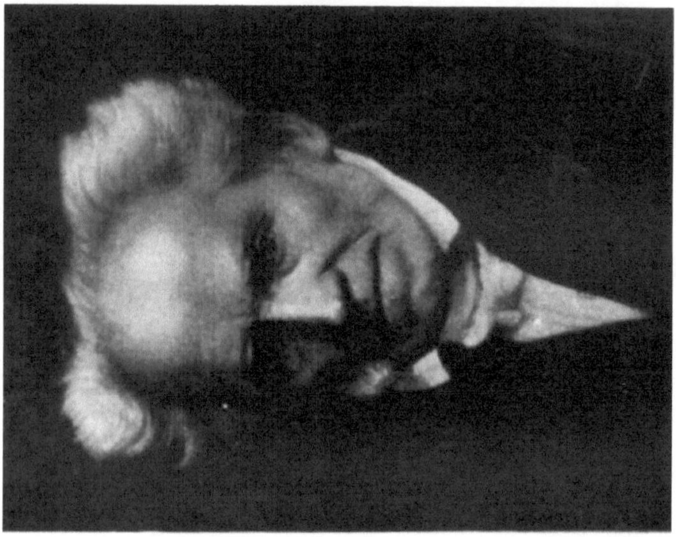

SCHOPENHAUER, PHILOSOPHER

(*See page* 200)

reduced, and *judgment is often poor* and erroneous owing to the absence of elements of contrast".

CHAS. K. MILLS (*Nervous System and its Diseases*, 1898) pointed out that in lesions of the frontal lobes, "mental symptoms of a peculiar character occur, such as mental slowness and uncertainty, want of attention and control, and *impairment of judgment and reason*".

P. W. MACDONALD (*Journal of Mental Science*, 1902) said: "Notwithstanding the intimacy, sympathy, and collaboration between the various sections of the grey cortex of the brain, there would still seem to be a consensus of opinion in favour of the theory that the finer reasoning processes of mental actions are localised in this pre-frontal region."

ALLEN STARR, who had studied the mental disturbances following disease of the frontal lobes, gave the summary of twenty-three cases in the *American Journal of Mental Science*, 1894. He laid great stress on the frontal brain being an inhibitory organ. He regarded it therefore as the seat of judgment and reason, the highest psychical manifestations. Through the loss of self-control, he said, the attention can no longer be fixed, and the patient can no longer follow the sequence of his ideas. He regarded the loss of attention as important. He said, "The form of mental disturbance in lesions of the frontal region does not conform to any type of insanity. It is rather to be described as a loss of self-control, and a subsequent change of character. This action of control implies a recognition of the importance of an act in connection with other acts—in a word, it involves judgment and reason, the highest mental qualities. *It seems probable that the processes involved in judgment and reason have, for their physical basis, the frontal lobes;* if so, the total destruction of these lobes would reduce man to the state of an idiot; while their partial destruction would be manifested by errors of judgment and reason of a striking character. One of the first manifestations would be a lack of that self-control which is a constant accompaniment of mental action, and which would be shown by an inability to fix the attention to follow a continuous train of thought, or to conduct intellectual processes. It is this very symptom that was present in one-half of the cases collected. It occurred in all forms of lesions—from injury by foreign bodies, from destruction by abscess, from compression by softening due to the pressure of tumours—and, therefore, cannot be ascribed to any one form of disease. It did not occur in lesions of other parts of the brain."

CHAPTER X

THE FRONTAL LOBES AND SPECIAL ABILITIES

Arithmetical Ability

Arithmetical ability is one of the capacities that cannot be explained by any process of development due to the struggle for existence, or to sexual selection. Yet, the arithmetical talent seems to be a special faculty of the human mind. Though all normal children can be taught to count, some learn quickly, others slowly. Some men take a delight in working out arithmetical problems, others have a distaste for them; and it often happens that those who are very skilful in solving such problems have no unusual ability for anything else.

There are two things necessary for an ability to reckon rapidly; a powerful memory for figures, and a real ability for calculating. The carrying out of long calculations in the mind depends, above all, on the accuracy of the memory over a sufficient length of time. The power to commit a group of objects, or a line of a dozen figures, rapidly to memory, and to call it up again instantly, depends on the ease and rapidity with which one can impress it on the mind; on the accuracy with which it is reckoned, and on the facility with which it can be reproduced. The ease and rapidity with which a number of objects can be impressed on the memory seem limited, in average persons, to about five at a glance. In regard to a special inclination for mathematics, and its relation to ability for calculation, and to other abilities likewise, great diversity is exhibited.

The possessors of this wonderful faculty generally come of obscure families who have never shown particular skill in arithmetic. Besides the capacity of keeping figures in memory and rapidly calculating, it is of importance that the reckoners should keep up the use of their talent; for, without practice, they seem to lose much of their facility.

In the *Lancet* of November 1922, V. Numair makes the assertion that calculating prodigies owe their powers, mainly, to early environment. This cannot be; for there are numerous cases on record of imbeciles, confined in institutions, who, from infancy—though the faculty of number is usually on a par with the lack of general intelligence in the mentally deficient—yet showed extraordinary abilities in this direction. That there must be an anatomically distinct brain centre for the formation and expression of figures is shown, also, by the numerous cases of aphasia (loss of articulate speech) recorded, in which the ability to calculate, and the expression of figures, were retained. Further, a patient may be word-blind (unable to read words), and yet be able to calculate and read figures. One more fact against the presumption of the environmental influence is that the great calculators showed precocity for figures, in some instances at three years of age; in others at six; and, most of them, before ten years of age.

Strange as the fascination for arithmetic seems, it becomes still more so when it is manifested at an age at which it is normally absent. Strangest of all is the union of ability with the inclination. Sir William Broadbent (*British Medical Journal*, 1907), gave a number of cases of London County Council schoolboys who could not learn to spell or read, but "did difficult sums in arithmetic".

A. Binet (*Psychologie des Grands Calculateurs*, 1894) had studied Inaudi and Diamandi, two arithmetical geniuses who were examined by the Academy of Science in Paris. I saw Inaudi in London. A line of figures, casually suggested by members of the audience, was multiplied by another line, and the product given with astonishing rapidity. The ciphers were written on a blackboard behind the performer, so that they could be read by the spectators, but not by Inaudi. Nevertheless, he was able to hold in his memory and repeat all the figures. In adding, he used to begin at the left side with the higher numbers. He dealt with the numbers as sounds: that is, they had to be repeated to him orally, whereas Diamandi regarded them as seen figures.

Arithmetical ability is not confined to Europeans. In the *Korea Magazine*, May 1917, was an account by W. Carl Rufus, Ph.D., of the case of An Myengwhan, a Korean lad 16 years of age, in the employ of the Land Investigation Bureau. He was described as a perfect human adding machine. He could add up twenty-five items of four figures each in seven seconds by mental calculation; and when using an abacus the time required by him in making the same addition was eight seconds. Frequently at night he saw columns of figures before his closed eyes.

B. Glanville Corney (*Lancet*, 1922) mentioned the case of a native Fijian boy, only 10 years of age, brought up in a remote inland village, with no opportunities to learn or practise figures; and another, a youth from another part of the Fijian Islands, aged about 18, brought up in similar circumstances. "Both these boys would multiply, add, subtract, or divide amounts comprising from seven to ten figures by a mental process, in less time than we could do the sums on a slate; and they never made a mistake, though we sometimes did."

To be able to learn to speak is undoubtedly a measure of the capacity of imbeciles; but speech may be freely exercised without the existence of any ability to count. This deficiency is universal, comprising all classes of imbeciles. The old legal definition of an idiot is "one who cannot count twenty pence". The greater number of idiots cannot count three; but (as I have said and shall now give examples) imbecile children are sometimes found who are wonderfully skilled in calculations of various sorts, though with no other ability.

L. Lotte (*L'Encéphale*, 1920): *A blind lightning calculator.* The case of a feeble-minded boy, completely blind, age 26, named Fleury. "He can give the square root of any number running into four figures in an average of four seconds; and the cube root of any number running into four figures in an average of four seconds; and the cube root of any number running into six figures in six seconds; he gave the cube root of 34,012,224 (324) in 11 seconds, and the cube root of 465,484,375 (775) in 13 seconds. These seem mere trifles, however, compared with the following: He was asked how many grains of corn there would be in any one of 64 boxes: with one in the first, two in the second, four in the third, eight in the fourth, and so on in succession. He gave the answers for the 14th (8,192), for the 18th (131,072), and the 24th 8,388,608) instantaneously; and he gave the figures for the 48th box (140,737,488,355,328) in six seconds. Further, on the request to give the total in all the boxes up to and including the 64th, he furnished the correct answer (18,446,734,073,709,551,615) in 45 seconds. Fleury can give the day for Easter in any year in the Gregorian and Julian calendars respectively, and simultaneously by some scheme equally original."

William McAlister (*Lancet*, 1922): A similar case of a congenital imbecile, practically blind, who never learned to read the Braille type, could not write, and did not know what spelling meant, yet possessed an extraordinary memory for facts and events, and never forgot the date of anything that had come within the scope of his personal experience. Equally striking was the ease with which he told the day of the week on which a particular date fell. "After a perfunctory handshake he asked: 'What is your birthday?' and was told 'the 15th May'. Immediately came the response, 'Your birthday this year was on a Monday'. He then inquired, 'How old are you?' and was told '34'. Without hesitation he remarked, 'You were born on May 15, 1888; that was a Tuesday. You had a birthday on Tuesday in 1894, 1900, 1906, and 1917. You will not again have a birthday on a Monday till the year 1933, and after that in 1939, 1944', etc."

A. Wizel (*Archiv. f. Psychiatrie*, 1904) described a phenomenal talent of counting in an imbecile: Sabina W., age 22, inmate of a hospital at Warsaw. The family had a special gift for music, but none for arithmetic. Patient was normal till 7, when she had severe epileptic fits, followed by unconsciousness lasting for several days, leaving her an absolute imbecile. When she was 11 she was mentally the equal of a child of 3. The epileptic seizures continued, though in a milder form, but they were followed by fits of violence. At the age of 22 she was still weak-minded. She could not tell how old she was, or how many brothers and sisters she had; she could not read or write, could not read figures; and could only talk on childish subjects. She had no affection for anybody, and could not keep herself clean. But she had remarkable faculty for arithmetic, being especially good at multiplication and division. She divided 576, 560, and 336 by 16, and 225 and 270 by 15, with astonishing quickness; yet she failed in simple addition and subtraction; giving often the right answers, but much more slowly. Sabina possessed another power rarely met with in ordinary people. Once Dr. Wizel asked her, "What is the product of 23 × 23?" She quickly gave 529, and added, "That comes to as much as 33 × 16 and 1". Dr. Wizel gave numerous other examples. It was difficult to get Sabina to explain by what processes she so rapidly got her answers; but one example may explain. Asked to calculate 45 × 18 she answered "810"; Dr. Wizel thought she multiplied 90 × 9.

E. J. Swift in his book *Psychology and the Day's Work*, mentions the following calculating memory wonder: A university student named Ruckle gave an exhibition before the Congress for Experimental Psychology at Giessen. He was able to learn 204 figures in thirteen minutes so that he could repeat them. Ruckle differed from Inaudi and Diamandi in having an exceptional memory for other things than figures and numbers. He could learn a series of nonsense-syllables in less than half the time usually required. With Ruckle, however, as with others, recall was not based on mere memory. He made use of various devices which gave the figures meaning. For example, he separated them into columns, and each column served as a unit; and in remembering long numbers he divided them into their prime factors. Further than this, his method was to change what he heard into visual images. Then, as he put it, he saw the numbers as clearly as though they were written on a blackboard.

Among great arithmetical prodigies are:

NICKOMACHOS, of Gerasa (ca. 30 A.D.), mentioned by Lucianus.
THOMAS FULLER (1710–90), the Virginian calculator.
JEDEDIAH BUXTON (1707–90), of Derbyshire, England.
ANDRÉ MARIE AMPÈRE (1775–1836), of Marseilles.
CARL FRIEDRICH GAUSS (1777–1855), of Brunswick.
RICHARD WHATELEY (1787–1863), Archbishop of Dublin.
ZERAH COLBURN (1804–40).
VITO MANGIAMELE (ca. 1837), of Sicily.
ZACHARIAS DAHSE (1824–61), of Hamburg.
C. GRANDMANGE (ca. 1852), of Paris, born without legs or arms.
HENRY MONDEAUX (1826–62).
GEORGE BIDDER (1806–76), engineer.
TRUMAN HENRY SAFFORD (born 1836), of the United States.

On the other hand, there are men with a congenital deficiency in the faculty of number, for example, Beethoven and George Combe. The latter said:

"Arithmetic has always been a profound mystery to me; and to master the multiplication table an insurmountable task. I could not tell how much eight times nine are without going to work circuitously, and reaching it by means of the tens; yet for seven years I studied arithmetic. The faculty in me is, in fact, idiotic. Were my other powers in like condition, I should be totally unfit for the ordinary business of life."

The following is a case of Head Injury, followed by Loss of the Faculty of Number.

Plate XXXI

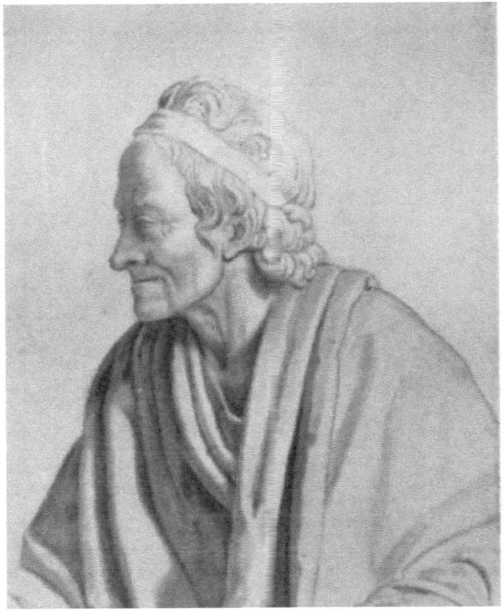

VOLTAIRE, PHILOSOPHER

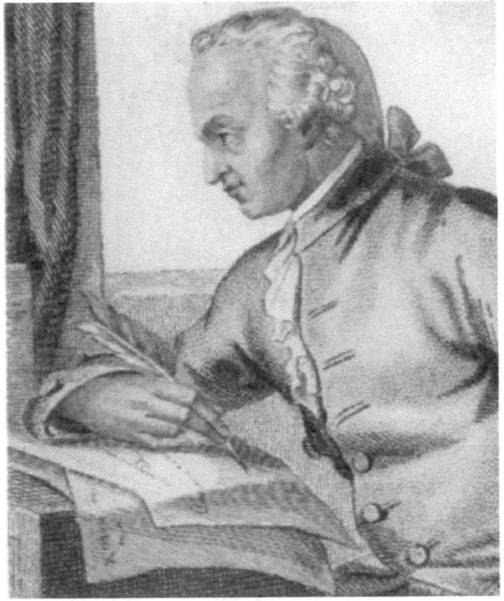

KANT, PHILOSOPHER

Notice the distance of the upper part of the forehead from the ear

(*See page* 260)

PLATE XXXII

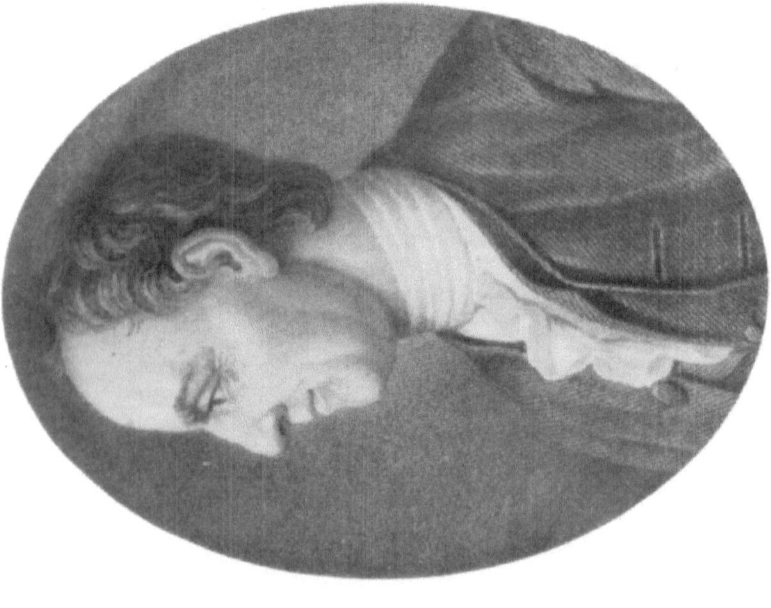

EULER, ARITHMETICAL GENIUS

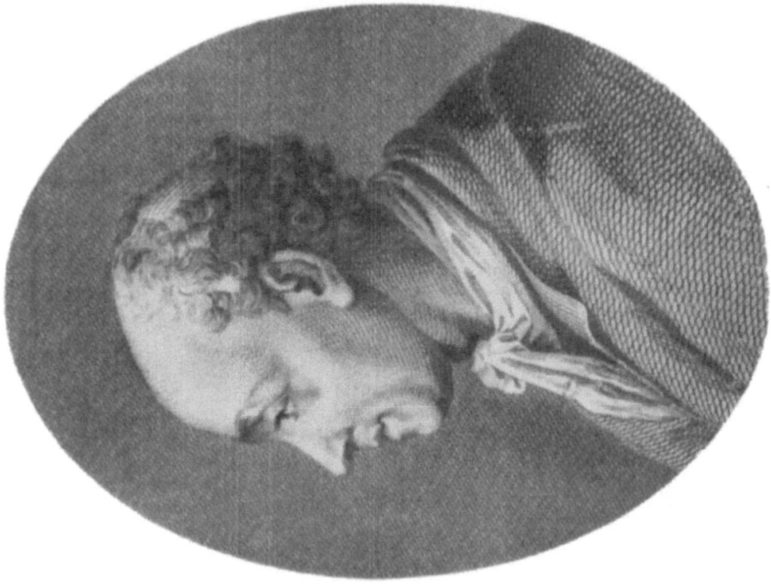

GESSNER, ARITHMETICAL GENIUS

(*See page* 203)

Plate XXXIII

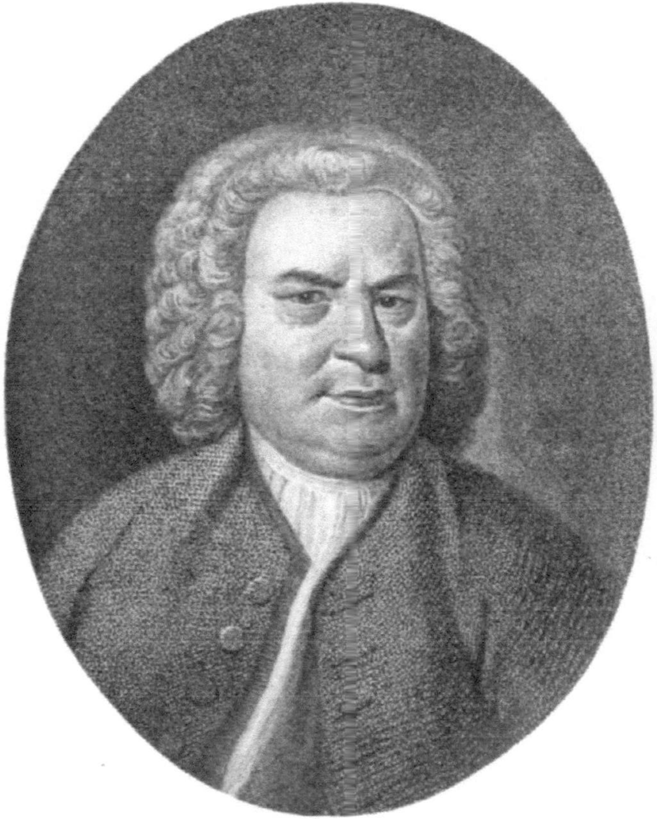

BACH, MUSICAL GENIUS

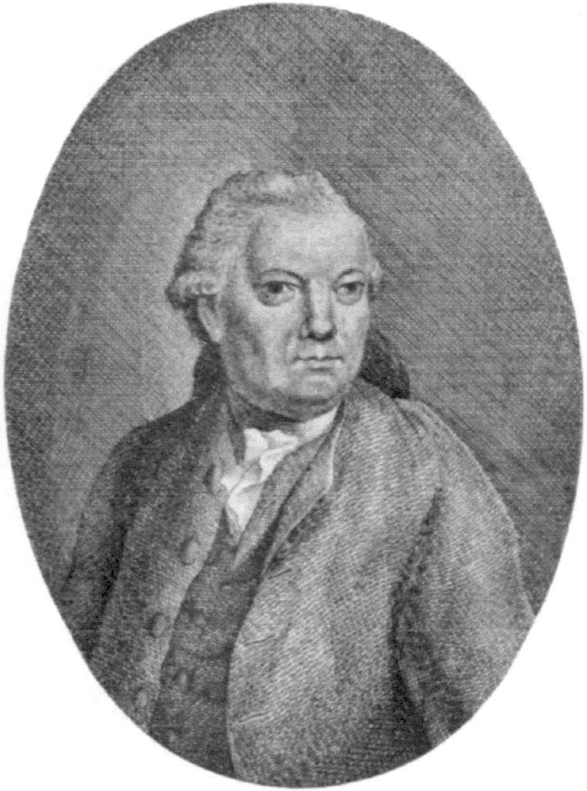

BENDA, MUSICAL GENIUS

(*See page* 212)

PLATE XXXIV

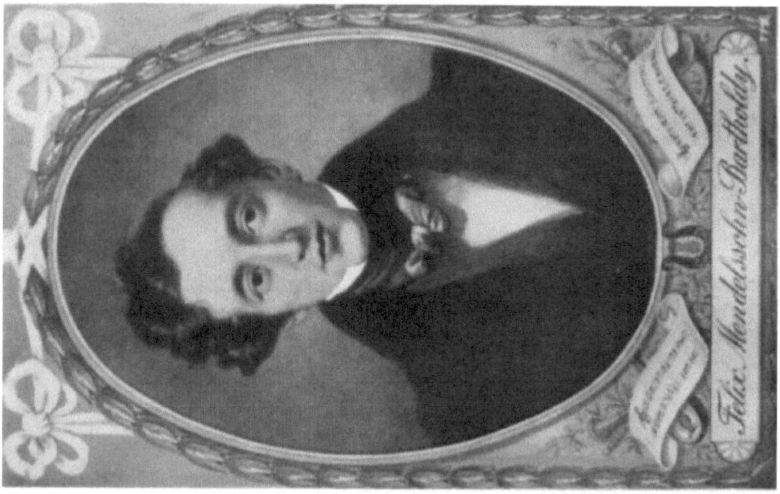

MENDELSSOHN

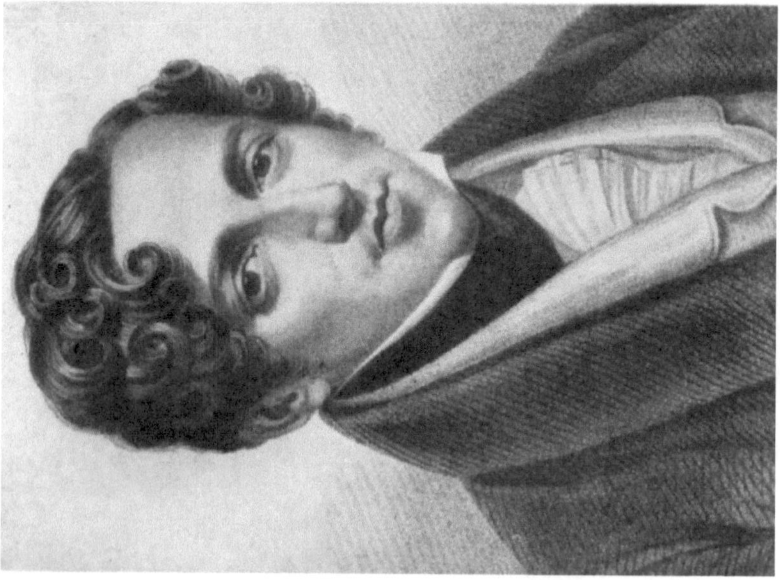

MEYERBEER

(*See page* 212)

K. RIEGER (*Centralblatt f. Nervenheilkunde*, 1887) showed, at a meeting of the Medical Association at Würzburg, a patient, Mr. Seybold, a sculptor of Carlstadt, who had received a fracture of the base of the skull in a railway accident. Patient spoke rather slowly, and was weaker in his memory than before the accident; but the chief symptom was that he had forgotten all ideas of figures, beyond 1, 2, and 3.

The following are cases of brain lesions followed by aphasia; but with the power of calculation, and the expression of numbers, retained.

Case of Aphasia with Retention of Expression of Figures

VOLLAND (*Münchener Medizinische Wochenschrift*, 1886): A farmer's son, age 15, had a fall which injured the scalp, but not the bone. When after several days he recovered consciousness, though he understood everything that was said to him, he could nevertheless only reply one word, "Anna", by speech or in writing. Yet he was able to count up to 100, to recite the multiplication table, and to add or subtract figures. He could write all figures, and calculate correctly on paper. Gradually, he acquired the power to speak whole sentences, but did not get on well at school except in arithmetic, in which he was equal to the best. Six years after the accident he was still somewhat aphasic, had attacks of giddiness, and slight ptosis. This case shows that the formation and expression of words must be anatomically separate from the formation and expression of figures.

Another Case of Aphasia with Retention of Expression of Figures

SCHRÖDER VAN DER KOLK (*Pathology and Therapeutics of Mental Disease*, p. 14): A tradesman came, conducted by his son, to obtain the doctor's advice. About half a year back the father had had an apoplectic attack of short duration, which left no paralysis; yet the memory for names or words had in a great measure vanished, so that he called objects by wrong names, and, for example, used the word "chair" when he meant a table. Yet he well knew the word "chair" was not the usual one, and he brought forward other words, until at last he came to "table", which word he then pronounced with great satisfaction. There was yet another suppression which the doctor had not previously observed. The patient was no longer able to read, although the sight was not impaired. On a large printed book being placed before the man, he distinguished the letters in it quite well, and spelt, for example, the word "towards", but he was not able to combine these letters into a word. The man had also lost the capacity of writing; so that he could no longer sign his name. But the most remarkable circumstance with this patient was that he could still—according to the assurance of his son—*keep his ledger, and reckon now as ever before.*

Other Cases of Aphasia with Retention of Expression of Figures

L. V. Marcé (*Gazette Médicale de Paris*, 1856):

Case 7. The patient could not write his name from memory, but wrote figures and solved complicated arithmetical exercises, always setting the figures in their proper places.

Case 11. Patient distinguished single letters quite well, but was no longer able to combine them into a word. He transcribed a word quite correctly, but could not write it when it was dictated to him. Yet he could write figures very well.

Otto Hebold (*Allg. Zeitschrift f. Psychiatrie*, 1894): H. G. had loss of speech, but could calculate correctly.

Pringle Morgan (*British Medical Journal*, 1896): Recorded a case in which the memory for words and letters was lost; but not that for figures, from which he inferred that there is not only a complete functional independence of these two faculties, but also an anatomical independence.

Heilly and Chantemesse (*Progrès Médical*, Vol. XI): A case of sensory aphasia with the power of calculation preserved. The authors mention that patient could play écarté correctly.

A. Chauffard (*Revue de Médecine*, 1881): Case of sensory

aphasia. Had a tendency to substitute numerals for words. His appreciation for music was well preserved, though he complained that he could not hear words.

DÉJERINE (*Comptes rendus des séances de la Société de Biologie*, 1892): Patient, although word-blind, could write as fluently as ever. He could copy, correctly, pages of manuscript; although he could not read a word he had written. He had also lost the power of reading musical notes; but he could still sing. He could read figures, and do mental calculations just as well as ever.

BRANDENBURG (*Graefe's Archiv. f. Ophthalmologie*, 1888): A hitherto healthy man had an apoplectic stroke, which made him temporarily aphasic. There was alexia, but no agraphia. The patient could write anything, but could not read, with the exception of figures, so that the reading of numbers was preserved.

M. LANNOIS (*Lyon Médical*, 1898): Patient, age 32, had been for three years in a condition of complete amnesia, with the exception of the memory for figures. He could not write spontaneously anything except figures, and calculation remained his only occupation.

JAMES HINSHELWOOD (*Lancet*, 1895): A teacher of languages, age 58, who had had of recent years a large amount of mental work, and before his present visual difficulties appeared, considerable mental worry and anxiety, found suddenly one morning that he could not read the exercises as usual. Greatly puzzled, he took up a printed book, and found that he could not read a single word. On examining his visual acuity, Dr. Hinshelwood found that he was unable to read even the largest letters of the test types. Patient informed him that he could see all the letters plainly and distinctly, but could not say what they were. What attracted special attention was the fact that the patient read at once the number standing at the top of each paragraph of the test types. On examining further, it was found that he did not experience the slightest difficulty in reading any number of figures quite fluently, and without making any mistakes whatever. He could read figures printed on the same scale as Jaeger No. 1, the smallest of the test types; and from other tests it was evident that there was no lowering of his visual acuity. The inability to read was thus manifestly not due to any failure of visual power, but to a loss of the visual memory for letters. The page of a printed book appeared to him exactly as it appears to a person who has never learned to read. He saw each individual character distinctly enough, but the character was no longer a visual symbol, as he no longer remembered any special significance attached to it. His difficulty with written characters was equally well marked. He could write with perfect fluency and ease to dictation, although afterwards he could not read what he himself had written. He spoke as fluently as ever. *Patient was tested further with large combinations of figures, and all these were read with the greatest fluency, and without hesitation whatever.*

Cases of arithmomaniacs—patients dominated by an irresistible impulse to count everything, and to make useless calculations—while otherwise of normal intellect and conduct, have been reported by TRÉLAT (*La Folie Lucide*); A. CULLÈRE (*Annales Médico-Psychologiques*, 1890); and LUDWIG BRUNS (*Neurologisches Centralblatt*, 1891).

All these facts make it highly probable that the memory for numbers and the calculating ability are inherent in the brain and must depend on a special centre in the frontal lobes. As Professor S. E. HENSCHEN has said (*Brain*, 1926): "The cases published show clearly that special centres exist for calculation, and that they are separated from those of language and music. These centres lie, however, *in the neighbourhood of those of language and music*, for there is often a disturbance of all three; but the centre for calculation is often preserved when the centres for language or music are destroyed."

MUSICAL ABILITY

It would be difficult to settle what are distinct talents or innate gifts; but it will scarcely be denied that the musical talent is one of them. Nevertheless, it is made up of a number of elements, of which the principal one is the sense of appreciation of tones. The appreciation of sounds, alone, is not music; for music is a harmonious arrangement of sounds. The "time" sense, among other factors, is required to appreciate it. That the capacity for music does not depend merely on acuity of hearing was proved by Beethoven, who produced, among other compositions, the *Ninth Symphony* and the *Mass in D* after he had become deaf. We must also distinguish between mere executants and composers. The latter require phantasy in addition to the other qualities which constitute musical ability.

In persons who, in common language, have no ear for music, there is not auditory deafness, but an inability of the nervous structure to appreciate the minute vibrations caused by the more subtle differences, in or among musical sounds; in other words, such people are tone-deaf. A man may be almost deaf, and yet appreciate and even compose music; while another may have a highly developed sense of hearing, and yet find music distressing. Undoubtedly musical ability is a complex faculty. Many cases have been noted in which this inherent power has become affected in brain disease, chiefly in lesions of the anterior portions of the temporal lobe adjoining the frontal; but I believe that certain of the elements of musical ability—such as appreciation of harmony and time—are intellectual processes—and must be in the frontal lobes.

In mental derangement the musical ability is often preserved. Sir JOHN BATTY TUKE had two lady patients who—though quite incoherent in speech—played with great accuracy on the piano; the one by ear, the other from written scores; although the latter was quite unable to read a book, and had not dressed herself for twenty years (*Journal of Mental Science*, 1891).

Memory of tune is often found among the feeble-minded. They readily acquire simple airs, and rarely forget them. The turn for music is quite disproportionate to their other mental faculties; and, not infrequently, those who cannot speak at all, can correctly hum tunes. This remarkable development of the musical sense in the feeble-minded is the more striking on account of the utter absence of any other evidence of artistic taste. A beautiful landscape, or a lovely picture, is utterly powerless to move them.

Sir Astley Cooper mentioned the case of a man very deaf from childhood, who, notwithstanding, appreciated harmony; this person played well on the flute, and performed with great success in concerts.

Darwin knew a child who loved music extremely, and could easily retain an air after hearing it sung distinctly, but whose organ of hearing was yet so imperfect that it was necessary to speak very loudly in addressing him.

Blind Tom (Thomas Wiggins), known throughout two continents for his wonderful musical genius, was little more than a child of feeble mind in all relations of life except that of music. He reproduced with an exactness little short of the marvellous what he had heard immediately before. But the wonder was, that once having reproduced the execution of a musical composition, he never afterwards lost memory of it. He also composed some pieces of his own. Beyond the sphere of music, he failed to rise above the intelligence of a child of six. His passion for music began when two years old, and he never lost it until a few days before he died, when he was stricken with apoplexy. In his retirement he spent eight hours of each day at the piano. The rest of his life was a blank. Having made fortunes for his owners and guardians, he died in 1908, in his sixtieth year. He was of the pure negro race, a slave born in Georgia. His mother was bought by Colonel James N. Bethune in 1850. At the time, she carried in her arms a babe, blind and so feeble, that in the sale the babe was thrown in with the mother. He was the wonder of America and Europe; and although he was almost an imbecile in everything but music, he showed in this extraordinary talent.

Dr. LANGDON DOWN had under his care an idiot boy who could tell the time—besides the words and number of nearly every hymn in *Hymns Ancient and Modern.* Another boy in his care, following a visit to the opera, would carry away a recollection of all the airs, and would hum and sing them correctly.

ESQUIROL, a century ago, called attention to the fact that even idiots without the power of speech could sing.

WILDERMUTH (*Allg. Zeitschrift f. Psychiatrie,* 1889) estimated that the musical capabilities are well developed in one-third of even badly speaking idiots; and that though first-class musicians predominated amongst normal children, second, third, and fourth-class musical capacity existed more frequently amongst idiots.

Music thus appears to be a rudimentary endowment demanding a much lower capacity than that of speech, and less liable to be destroyed in mental decay.

The appreciation of musical sounds appears much earlier in life than the appreciation of words. Children sing, perceive, and enjoy music, before they speak. Dvořák's son manifested great delight at the sound of music when three months old, and retained the memory of melodies when one year old. Musical prodigies are numerous. No examples are needed. That with the gift of music there is also a remarkable memory for it is shown by Mozart, who, after hearing but once the *Miserere* of Allegri, wrote it out from memory.

That speech is unnecessary for the learning of melodies is also evidenced by birds—for instance, the bullfinches. Moreover, that the musical capacity is independent of the speech centres is shown by the loss of musical perception and of the ability to sing, without the simultaneous loss of speech and the power of understanding spoken words. It is only within the last few decades that attention has been drawn to the fact that the musical capacity may be lost from various pathological causes; and, further, that musical aphasia may occur either in conjunction with ordinary aphasia or independently of it.

Cases are on record in which the patients, though "word-blind", still retained the power of reading musical notes. In other cases there is loss of the visual memory for musical notes, though they can read words. The patients can see the notes, as usual; but they no longer have the faintest idea of their significance. They may be able to read the words of a song, but can no longer read the accompanying music.

Similarly, there may be deafness for spoken words, without deafness for musical tones, or the reverse; or there may be complete deafness for both. The notes are heard, but simply as sounds, the patients being unable to assign to them their position in the musical scale.

J. B. Bouillaud (*Bulletins de l'Académie de Médecine*, Vol. XXX), almost a century ago, made the observation on a patient, age 50, who had lost the memory for words almost entirely, and could speak and write but little, that he could compose an original tune, listen carefully when it was played to him, and sing the words correctly to the accompaniment.

J. P. Falret, in 1867, called attention to the fact that many aphasics who are unable to speak are still able to sing; some without words, but others with the words that they are unable to speak.

L. G. Ballet, in 1886, described musical aphasia, agraphia, and musical deafness.

A. Knoblauch (*Deutsches Archiv. f. Klinische Medizin*, 1888), who introduced the term "amusia" for the loss of the musical

Plate XXXV

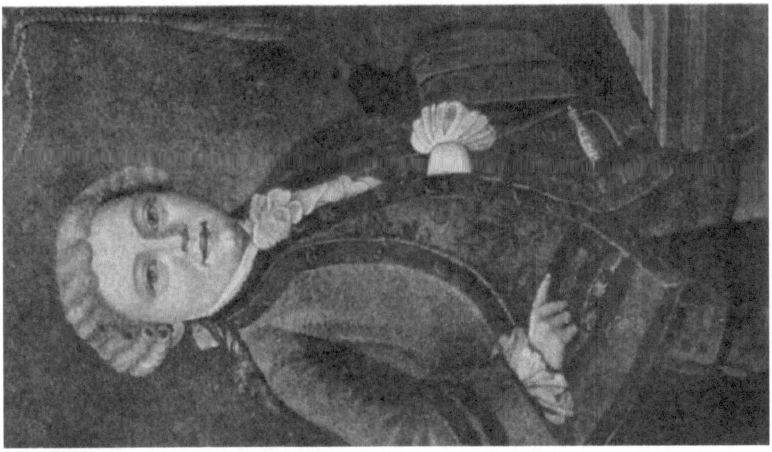

MOZART

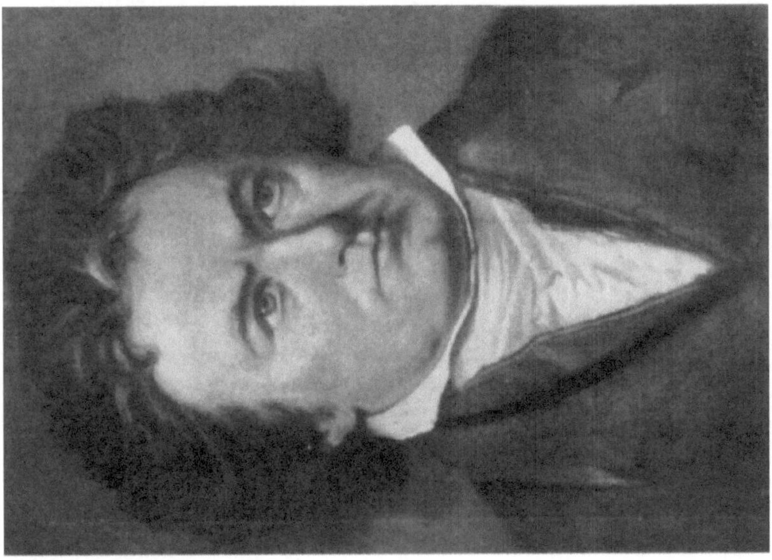

BEETHOVEN

(*See page* 212)

Plate XXXVI

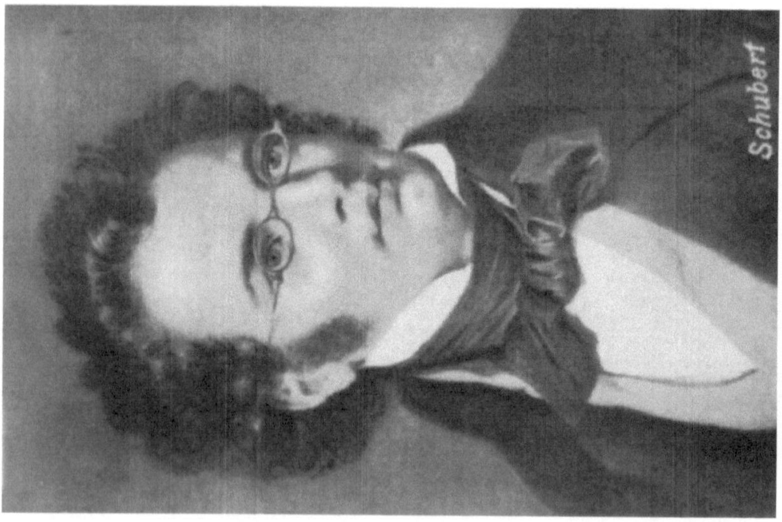

SCHUBERT

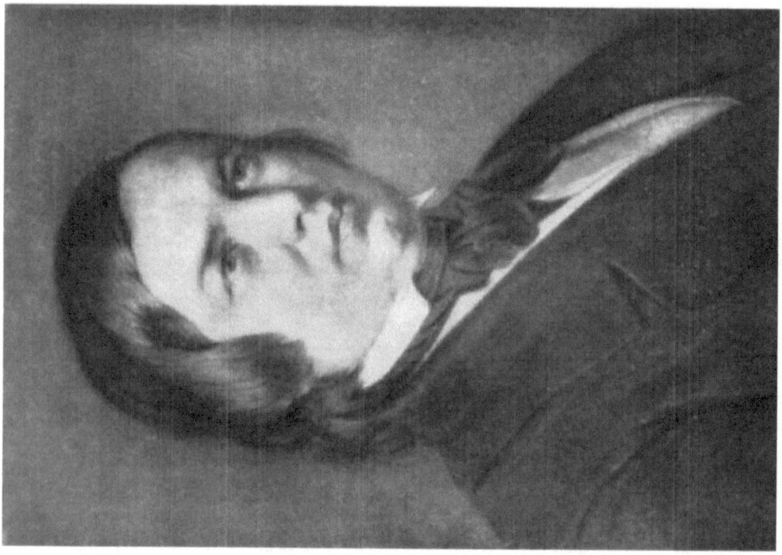

SCHUMANN

(*See page* 212)

PLATE XXXVII

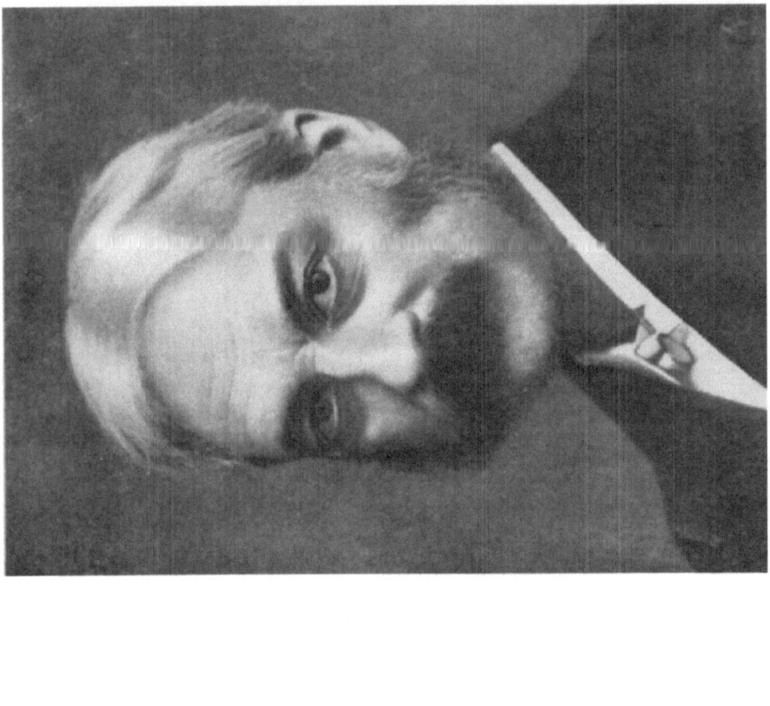

ANDREW LANG
Acknowledged to have no "ear for music" in a letter to the author

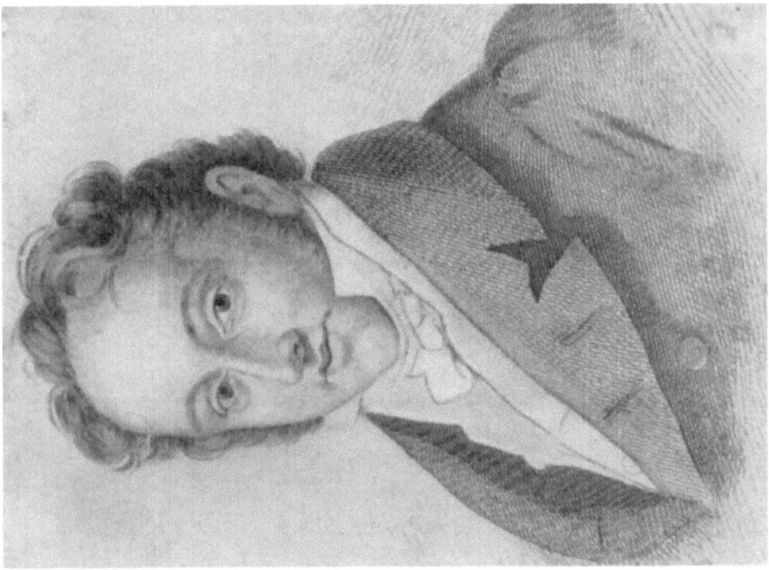

ROSSINI, MUSICAL GENIUS

PLATE XXXVIII

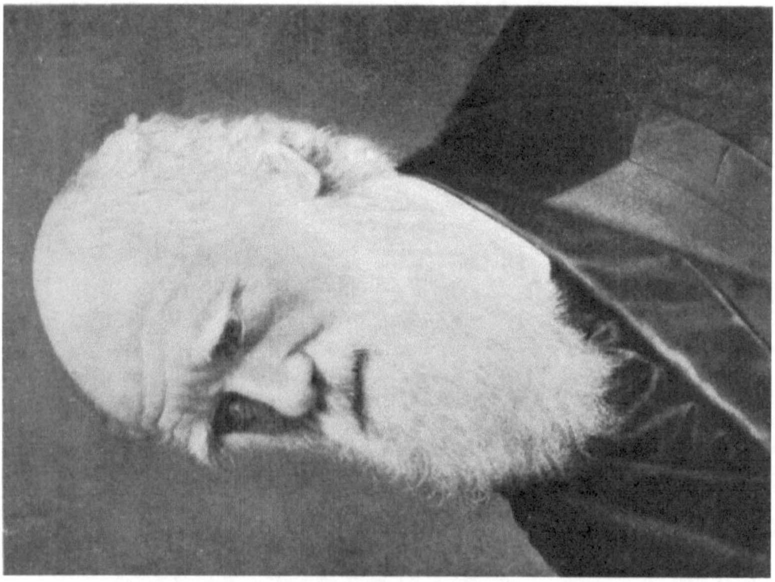

CHARLES DARWIN
"No ear for music"

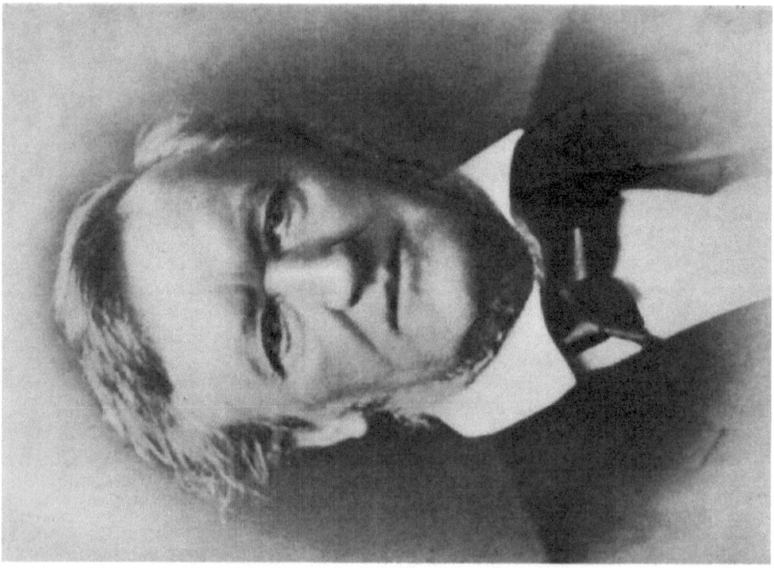

RICHARD WAGNER, MUSICAL GENIUS

sense, cites the case of a little girl, Lizette S., age six, who had right hemiplegia with aphasia. At first the child could not speak at all. Later she said "mamma", and apparently repeated a few words. She could sing the song *Weisst Du wie viel Sternlein stehen*, etc., but she could not recite the text of the song, or speak voluntarily single words of the same.

H. Oppenheim (*Charité Annalen*, 1888) found that many aphasics retain their musical faculty, and are able to recognise and appreciate melodies and music after they have lost the power to understand language, and are able to sing, sometimes even with words they cannot speak; others could read or write notes, though they could not read or write words. He published clinical notes of seventeen cases of aphasia, in which the musical faculty had been the subject of careful inquiry. The general result of these observations was that the musical faculty survived the loss of speech in aphasia; though in some patients the other mental powers were evidently injured. After the memory for melodies, the memory for numbers was found to be the best preserved. One patient, though he could not read ordinary letters, and could not write to dictation, nor copy writing properly, could quite well read and copy musical notes, or write them to dictation.

L. v. Frankl-Hochwart (*Deutsche Zeitschrift f. Nervenheilkunde*, 1891) studied the injury to the capacity for musical expression in five cases of aphasia. In all of these the musical power was less injured than that of speech. Some of them could sing words which they could not speak. Two could play from the music-book, one the violin, the other the piano, but they could not sing from it.

Brazier cites some cases in which there was no aphasia, but the patients could not distinguish musical airs with which they were usually familiar.

Edgren, of Stockholm, published in the *Deutsche Zeitschrift f. Nervenheilkunde*, 1894, a collection of 52 cases of aphasia without amusia, and of pure amusia without aphasia; showing the anatomical independence of the centres for speech and appreciation of tones.

Bianchi (op. cit.) published the case of a man suffering from complete aphasia who was able to sing popular Neapolitan songs.

E. G. Lasègue had an aphasic and agraphic patient who could write down a composition with ease after hearing it played.

P. Blaikie Smith (*British Medical Journal*, 1897): A seaman, age 51, though he could hear, did not understand what was said to him. He acquired lip-reading. His remarks were always short, and every now and then he would misapply a word. He could name objects correctly and without hesitation. His musical faculty was impaired. Well-known airs, such as the National Anthem, he failed to recognise. His intelligence seemed unaffected. He recovered from the auditory aphasia first, from the amusia much later.

Case of Temporal Lesion with Sensory Aphasia and Tone Sense Preserved

Ludwig Bruns (*Allg. Zeitschrift f. Psychiatrie*, 1892) showed, at the meeting of the German Alienists at Hanover on May 1, 1891, the brain of a musician with sensory aphasia who had not lost the tone sense. There was softening of the first temporal convolution, with the exception of the anterior part.

Another Case of Aphasia—Musical Sense Preserved

Bernard (*De l'Aphasie*, Paris, 1889): Lady, music teacher, age 45, had an apoplectic stroke, became hemiplegic on the right side and aphasic; but recovered the power of speech gradually, though she now expressed herself with difficulty. Yet she sang the tune *La dame blanche vous regarde* with the correct melody, pronouncing every word distinctly, and other tunes besides. She was not word-deaf, and could read a few sentences from a newspaper. She could read the title of music-scores; yet not the actual score. Of this she could not read a single note. Of all pieces of music put before her, she could read the title, but failed with the notes. Post-mortem, a long strip of the convolutions within the *fossa Sylvii* was found destroyed.

Case of Frontal Lesion—Aphasia—Musical Sense Preserved

FINKELNBURG (*Berliner Klinische Wochenschrift*, 1870): A professional violin player, after an apoplectic stroke, lost considerably the memory of names of objects, and more so of abstract ideas. He could still play the violin by ear as ably as before, but not from notes, which he constantly mistook. He could no longer write notes without making mistakes. Another stroke deprived him of speech altogether, of the power of writing, and the ability to read notes. Post-mortem, the cortical layer of the *island of Reil* and the neighbouring parts were found softened.

Other observers of the independence of the tone sense are STUMPF, STRICKER, WALLASCHEK, BLOCQ, BRISSAUD, DONATH, WÜRTZEN, MARINESCO, LICHTHEIM, KAHLER, PICK, WERNICKE, ANTON, LARINOW, HUGHLINGS JACKSON, GOWERS, GRASSET, and HALLOPEAU.

Some observers assume that amusia may be situated in the anterior part of the first temporo-sphenoidal convolution, in front of Wernicke's area for word-deafness; but I am inclined, from a study of the evidence, to seek the centre for the appreciation of the relation of tones in the small anterior convolutions within the folds of the fissure of Sylvius that lie between the inferior frontal and superior temporal convolutions. Its definite localisation, however, must be the subject of future investigation. Here, we must content ourselves in bringing the literature concerning this problem, and records of cases, together.

PAUL FLECHSIG discovered the end stations of the cochlea nerves in this region; and this localisation harmonises with Ferrier's observations.

PROBST (*Archiv. f. Psychiatrie*, 1899) located the tone-centre in the most anterior parts of the left temporal lobe.

URQUHART (*Journal of Mental Science*, 1904) found that the

lesion, in a case of loss of musical capacity, was at the tip of the temporal lobe.

Bronislawski (*Contribution à l'étude de l'amusie et de la localisation des centres musicaux.* Thèse de Bordeaux, 1900) located the sensory centre for music in the anterior two-thirds of the superior temporal convolution and the anterior half of the middle one; and the motor centre for singing in the second left frontal convolution. He mapped out several other centres for the different varieties of musical capacity, very much as others have located the various forms of aphasia all over the brain. *He had even a special centre for wind instruments!*

Professor S. E. Henschen, of Stockholm (*Brain*, 1926), stated that "the power of playing musical instruments, and its pathological form *musical apraxia*, may not be localised in a constant and circumscribed cortical centre, but *may be represented in different localities according to different instruments*". This does not seem to me probable. Professor Henschen examined one hundred cases of amusia, and found singing lost in lesions at the base of the third left frontal convolutions in front of Broca's centre; and instrumental incapacity (instrumental amusia) in lesions of base of second right frontal.

K. Mendel found the same.

Mercier and Newington (*Journal of Mental Science*, 1907) argued that the tone sense cannot be localised.

L. Mann, H. Forster, Rohardt (*Neurologisches Centralblatt*, 1919) cite several *cases of amusia* in lesions of *right frontal lobes.* Musical appreciation was retained, but the capacity of reproduction and production was lost. Here is one of them: Soldier, 24 years of age, injured by shell splinter on right side of forehead adjoining the temple. Was operated. Visible scar left. Formerly musical; now, could neither sing nor whistle a tune, mixed up notes hopelessly. There was no aphasia.

Case of Head Injury with Loss of Musical Capacity

A. Kast (*Deutsches Archiv. f. Klinische Medizin*, 1888): A youth, age 15, fell from a cart, and struck his head against the wheel. The accident was followed by loss of consciousness, lasting several hours. On restoration to consciousness, it was found that the right side of the body was paralysed, and that—though he seemed to comprehend what was said to him—he could not utter a word. The paralysis slowly disappeared. At the end of two months the aphasia had altered its character. The boy was no longer unable to speak, but had completely lost the artistic use of his vocal cords; though, prior to his accident, he was a distinguished member of a choral society. He sang discordantly, and quite out of tune, and could not correctly follow the lead of another singer.

Case of Frontal Injury with Loss of Musical Capacity

G. A. Königsfeld of Aix-la-Chapelle (*Zeitschrift f. Physiologie*, Heidelberg, 1876): J. Trump, a singer, age 18, received a kick

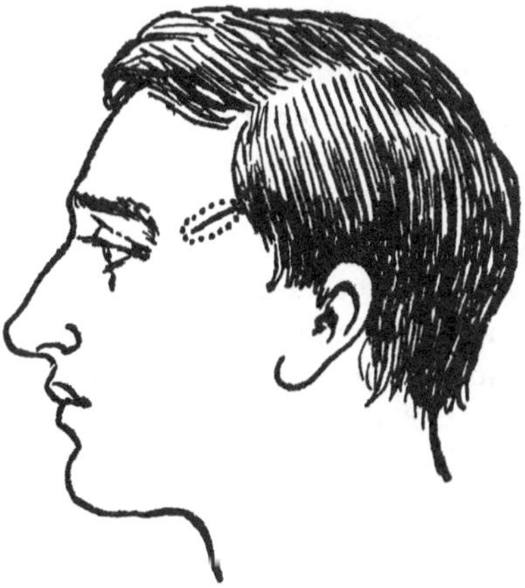

Plate XXXIX.—illustration to case of head injury
(J. Trump)
Lost his memory for music

from a horse, resulting in a fissured fracture of the frontal bone, the fissure running from the outer corner of the left eyebrow, upwards along the borderline of forehead and temple. The particles of bone were pressing on the brain, and the brain was contused. The wound suppurated, but got well after surgical treatment, a broad, deep scar being left. The patient had not suffered in intellect after his recovery, but *had lost the memory of all the tunes he formerly knew.* (See Illustration.)

Cases of Frontal Injury, with Loss of Tone Sense

J. G. EDGREN (*Hygeia*, 1894): The patient, age 34, knocked the side of his forehead against a lamp-post on August 31, 1890, and fell to the ground. He complained of headache afterwards, of imperfect sight, vomiting, difficulty of speech, and abnormality in the sense of taste. On September 17th, patient came home, after a visit to several concert halls, and declared he could not make out the music. He had intentionally tried several places; but though he could hear the music, it did not sound as usual, but more like an indefinite noise, so that he could not make out the melody. The reply his wife gave him he failed to understand, and he spoke no more for two days. On September 20th he began to speak again, but in so confused and disconnected a manner, that it was almost impossible to understand him. Admitted to hospital on September 23rd he was word-deaf. He could hear when someone was speaking to him, but without understanding the words spoken. Written communications he apprehended immediately; and he could still calculate. He heard equally well on both sides; he could hear the ticking of a watch at seven centimetres distance. His sense of smell was reduced; he could not smell spirits or vinegar. On October 5th his sense of smell and taste were perfectly normal. His defects were, therefore, only temporary, with the exception of his tone-deafness. He left the hospital on November 3rd. *Before the accident he had a good musical ear, which had now vanished, so that orchestral music was to him mere noise; he could not distinguish a waltz from a polka or march.* He used to sing to his children, but now, when attempting to do so he failed, and lost the melody. On March 17, 1893, he was readmitted for bronchitis. Intellect quite normal; no traces of aphasia; no word-deafness; only tone-deafness. He died. The post-mortem examination revealed destruction of the anterior two-thirds of the first temporal convolution, and the anterior half of the second temporal convolution of the left hemisphere, adjoining the frontal lobe.

Case of Head Injury with Temporary Loss of Musical Capacity

THOMAS D. SAVILL (*Clinical Lectures on Neurasthenia*, 1908): Mrs. Z., age 41, a professional singer and pianist, was struck severely on the left temple by falling glass from a seventh-floor window. She complained of loss of memory, confusion of thought, and complete inability to sing or play the piano. Though remembering ordinary matters well enough, she found herself utterly unable to read a single note of music, or to recognise delicate shades of intonation. At the time of the injury there had been a good deal of swelling and bruising over the left temple; but no fracture anywhere. Extreme tenderness continued. The loss of memory for musical signs persisted for over a year.

Case of Fronto-Temporal with Loss of Musical Faculty

FRANK HAY (*Journal of Mental Science*, Vol. XII): Patient, a musician, suffering from epilepsy, became aphasic, and lost the musical faculty as well. He could not be induced to sing, though formerly a member of a church choir. His humming and whistling were only in a monotone; and never in the nature of a tune. The autopsy revealed the tip of the temporo-sphenoidal lobe disorganised, and exposed a cavity which entered the fissure of Sylvius, and laid bare the insula and anterior extremity of the operculum.

L. WITHNEY (*Worcester Hospital Papers*, 1912–13): Case of tumour (a large endothelioma) of frontal lobes in a musician who had lost his musical capacity.

Congenital deficiency of the musical faculty may be seen in the portraits of Charles Darwin and Andrew Lang (see Illustrations). There is a difference, too, in the innate qualities of a musical executant and a musical composer.

There are other innate abilities which could be demonstrated to have definite relations to the brain—such as the ability for construction, i.e. manual dexterity—but these must be left to future investigators to explore.

CHAPTER XI

LESIONS OF THE FRONTAL LOBES FOLLOWED BY EXALTATION AND MORAL DEGENERATION

The Frontal Lobes and Mental Exaltation

It has already been demonstrated that any condition leading to hyperaemia of the frontal lobes causes an increased activity of the mental processes of perception, association, and reproduction. The patient forms numerous plans and projects, has a rapid flow of ideas, and, through the stimulation of the speech centre, is loquacious; but his stream of talk and ideas is perfectly coherent. It is only in the advanced stage that he may become incoherent. The other lobes of the brain being unaffected, but deprived of the control of the intellect, manifestations of the natural feelings and animal spirits occur, leading to childishness and childish actions. There is an increased muscular activity, unmeaning gaiety, peculiar hilarity, and tendency to jest, and there may be actual exaltation. The patient is free from hallucinations, knows his surroundings, and a chance observer might fail to recognise anything abnormal in him. The perfect health and general well-being of these patients renders them joyous, talkative, satisfied with themselves, and content with others. Natural dispositions, such as hope, pride, and ambition, in addition to the powers of the imagination, are stimulated to excess as the disease progresses; delusions of grandeur and of vanity, of increased wealth, power, and importance, may develop, followed later by confusion and disorientation, until finally all the ideas are affected, and chronic dementia is the result.

Both in functional and organic lesions of the frontal lobes, there is one characteristic that never occurs in lesions of other parts of the brain, that is, *the patient has no anxiety as to his condition*; on the contrary, frequently there is a feeling of joy, as seen in laughter and play, and general optimism—a mental condition called *euphoria* is present; while posterior lesions (parietal and occipital), as was shown in Chapter VI, give rise generally to low spirits, depression, apprehensiveness, and disturbances of sensation. In the one there is an excess, and in the other a diminution, of mental and muscular activity. The euphoria of frontal lesions is not based on delusions, but is absolutely free from any motive. It is, also, in sad contrast to the seriousness of the patient's condition.

> Temporary depression may precede the maniacal attack, from a vague consciousness of an approaching mental disturbance. A temporary state of depression may also follow the attack, in consequence of the exhaustion after the excessive mental and physical activity, and partly from the recollection of the mental illness and a reflection on the consequences of the many foolish things said and done. Such depression is, under the circumstances, perfectly natural, and should not be mistaken for "melancholia".

The patient's stream of talk, in the early stage of mania, is perfectly coherent; but it is not always refined, owing to the loss of inhibitory power over the propensities. Consequently, the patient may show erotic passion, or he may steal—if there is an inclination to it normally; but, even then, it is not done from a blind impulse, but from a desire to do mischief for the fun of the thing. This desire to do mischief for a companion's amusement may prove troublesome; but it is easily controlled by judicious management, and need not be regarded as dangerous.

Frequently, there is to be observed an inclination to

witticism, joking, punning—a state called moria—which, also, does not occur in lesions of other parts of the brain.

Professor Colin, of Val-de-Grâce, published in 1878 a paper on "General Paralysis", in which he declared that a lesion of the frontal lobes of the brain may become the starting-point of dementia paralytica (in which disease *exaltation* is the most marked mental symptom) by extension of what is at first a focal area.

Meynert (*Erkrankungen des Vorderhirns*, 1884) held that in mental derangements in which exaltation forms a prominent symptom, the frontal lobe is the affected part; not so in derangements in which depression is the leading characteristic.

A. Voisin (*Traité de la Paralysie Générale des Aliénés*, Paris, 1879) assumed a centre of exaltation—*centre de grandeur*—in the frontal brain.

J. B. F. Baillarger (*Annales Médico-Psychologiques*, 1881) published six cases of "ambitious delirium", i.e. mental exaltation, with focal lesions in the frontal lobes.

Pierre Marie (*Archives de Neurologie*, 1899) observed that "depressive or expansive religious systematised delusions are often noted in early psycho-motor disturbances" in the ascending frontal convolutions.

Tilney and Riley (*Form and Functions of the Central Nervous System*, 1921) recorded *changes in the personality* in lesions of the frontal lobes.

F. Obernier (*Ziemssen's Handbuch*, Vol. XI) considered exaltation to be one of the symptoms of tumours of the frontal lobes.

M. Jastrowitz (*Deutsche Medizinische Wochenschrift*, 1888) noticed in tumours of the frontal lobes a peculiarly cheerful excitement—hilarity and witticism—which was retained, sometimes, even on the operating table until the application of the anaesthetic. He observed, also, that the patient was given to grimaces.

In connection with this observation by Jastrowitz, I may mention an early experience of my own, when clinical assistant to Professor Krafft-Ebing in Vienna. We had a patient, a young man, who was to be operated on for tumour of the right frontal lobe. Before the operation the patient asked me: "Is it true, doctor, that you are going to cut my head open, wash it in an antiseptic, and put it back again?" I replied, "If we were to do that you might lose your head"; when the patient remarked: "Mother says there would not be much lost."

ALFRED GORDON (*Journal of American Medical Association*, 1907): J. M. H., age 34, "when asked where he was, replied 'In Paradise'. Every act and word expressed enchantment. He would joke with strangers, and expressed pleasure at anything offered him. Any article of food tasted delicious." Post-mortem, was found haemorrhage in left frontal lobe.

ERICH FEUCHTWANGER (*Die Funktionen des Stirnhirns*, 1922) had a large number of cases of lesions of the frontal lobes, in which the symptoms were joyful excitation, optimism, humour and wit, and active phantasy. *Two cases had laughing fits, and all seemed jollier than before their illness.*

CHURTON described at a meeting of the *Leeds and West Riding Medico-Chirurgical Society*, 1901, cases of frontal lesion that had come under his observation, and said the symptoms were: simple automatism, curious acts and mistimed humour, whimsical conduct, distorted memory.

H. OPPENHEIM (*Charité Annalen*, Vol. X, and *Archiv. f. Psychiatrie*, 1890) gave quite a number of cases of frontal tumour with *abnormal witticism and humorous remarks.*

L. BRUNS (*Deutsche Medizinische Wochenschrift*, 1892) also observed in frontal tumours, play with words—punning—and witticism. WILLIAMSON (*Brain*, 1896) quoted fifty cases of this kind.

A. RICHTER (*Allg. Zeitschr. f. Psychiatrie*, 1883) and KNÖRLEIN observed grimaces.

BRAMANN (*Archiv. f. Klinische Chirurgie*, Vol. XIV) described a case of abnormal cheerfulness in which, post-mortem, a tumour was found occupying almost the entire right frontal lobe.

GALAVIELLE and VILLARD (*Archives de Neurologie*, 1895) mention a case in which the whole left frontal lobe was occupied by a sarcoma, and in which the symptoms were aboulia, lack of interest, and diminution of intelligence. Patient spoke only "sottises".

P. E. Nunez (*L'Encéphale*, 1926) reviewed the literature dealing with the symptomatology of frontal lobe tumours, and described two cases of his own. He arrived at the conclusion that in the early stages of new growths, the most striking of the mental changes is "*hyperexcitation of the imagination*, which overrides the other faculties such as memory and attention, and often leads to an *irresistible optimism*. This latter gives place to a condition of psychical inhibition, somnolence, despondency, dullness, and stupor."

F. Lallemand (*Recherches Anat.-Patholog. sur l'Encéphale*) had a patient, Jean Bailly, age 60, who after some illtreatment by soldiers, had several paralytic seizures which passed off. Coincidently, his character changed. He developed an excessive hopefulness, a blind belief in obtaining a considerable fortune, and planned great enterprises. One characteristic deformity was observed; his mouth was drawn up on the right side. Post-mortem, a tumour was found, the size of a large egg on the posterior surface of the right frontal lobe.

V. Magnan (*Revue Mensuelle de Médecine et de Chirurgie*, 1879) reported a case of exaltation in which, post-mortem, a tumour was found in the ascending frontal convolution, about its middle third.

Castan and Lejonne (*Revue Neurologique*, 1901): A woman age 33 was admitted into the Salpêtrière with optic neuritis. Had Jacksonian epilepsy, and a peculiar mental disturbance. Suffering at the commencement of her illness from apathy and torpor, probably due to cerebral compression, she now passed into a state of high spirits, looking happy, and smiling when spoken to, complaining no longer, and showing signs of good humour and good appetite. Her intelligence seemed a little blunted, and *she laughed at almost anything which was said to her*, and exhibited little initiative or volition of her own. Her recollection of things said to her was poor. Her habits remained neat and clean, and she was free from dementia. A somnolent state succeeded the euphoria, lasting three months. The necropsy revealed a large cystic tumour, involving the posterior two-thirds of the left ascending frontal convolution.

L. Piqué (*Soc. de Chirurgie*, 1910): H., age 15, fell from a train, sustaining a comminuted fracture of right frontal lobe. Three months later developed *excessive gaiety, laughing incessantly.*

Case of Exaltation and Loss of Moral Sense

Charles W. Burr (*Journal of American Medical Association*, 1907): A woodworker, age 35, had his left frontal bone fractured in a railway accident. In a few weeks he became grandiose, careless as to money, and *obscene.*

Burr mentioned several other cases of apparently focal lesions, but gave no details as to their locality.

Cases of Frontal Lesion with Exaltation

Marandon de Montyel (*Annales Médico-Psychologiques*, 1877): In a patient suffering from *délire des grandeurs*, there was found, post-mortem, inflammatory adhesions of the meninges to the ascending frontal convolution.

Krafft-Ebing (*Traumatic Insanity*, Erlangen, 1868): G. B., age 29, farmer, fell from his carriage on the left side of the vault of the skull. He developed mania of *exaltation.* Death six years after the accident, when two sequestrae of bone were found in left ascending frontal convolution.

L. Marchand (*Soc. Anat.*, 1905): Patient hit by stone when four years old. Suffered from exaltation delirium from 15th year till death at 63. Post-mortem, softening of ascending frontal convolution.

Mendel (quoted by Paul Guder, *Geistesstörungen nach Kopfverletzungen*, 1886): Man, 36 years old, good history, was hit with a pistol on top of head. Scar two and a half inches long at sagittal suture, parallel with coronal suture. Paresis of arm, aphasia, exaltation. Post-mortem, the cranium was found thickened in the region mentioned, with exostoses; blood-extravasation, with pseudo-membrane internally.

Case of Frontal Lesion with Exaltation and Euphoria

V. MAGNAN (*Revue Mensuelle de Médecine et de Chirurgie*, 1878): The patient, a butcher, age 50, showed a few days before admission excessive activity in making exalted plans, and was possessed by an *abnormal cheerfulness and optimism*. Post-mortem, a symmetrical lesion was found in the middle three-fifths of each ascending frontal convolution; the lower congestion extending to half the middle and lower frontal convolutions.

F. X. DERCUM (*Journal of Nervous and Mental Disease*, 1910): M. S., age 32, merchant. "The patient's answers to questions are somewhat variable, and he is at times distinctly confused. He smiles readily, and seems quietly pleased. *He manifests no anxiety as to his condition*. He asks no questions." A huge tumour was removed from the frontal lobe. Patient died shortly afterwards.

D. CAMPBELL (*Monatsschrift f. Psychiatrie u. Neurologie*, 1910): "Patient, 37 years old, conscious of his surroundings, gave a correct account of his past history, but confabulated when interrogated about recent events, had no sense of time, did not know recent dates, was indifferent as to his condition, cheerful, witty, easily irritated, but quiet when left alone." Post-mortem, a tumour was found involving both frontal lobes.

GORDON BLACK (*British Medical Journal*, 1901) gave the case of a man whose mental symptoms commenced with forgetfulness and blundering at work, followed by loss of curiosity and interest in anything. As regards memory, replies to questions were normal, but "*gruffly humorous*". Post-mortem, a sarcoma was found as large as an orange, compressing both pre-frontal lobes.

Other cases of frontal tumours with exaltation and euphoria were observed by:

Bruns.	Eulenburg's Realencyclopaedie, 1895.
Siemens.	Berliner Klinische Wochenschrift, 1888.
J. B. F. Baillarger.	Annales Médico-Psychologiques, 1881.

Targoula.	Annales Médico-Psychologiques, 1890.
Thomas Lyle.	Journal of Mental Science, 1880.
Girot.	Société de Neurologie, 1925.
Vigouroux & Herisson-Lapane.	Bull. Soc. Clin. de Méd. Mentale, 1912.

Henri Baruk, op. cit.; Clouston, Raymond, Obernier, Peltavy.

Symptoms of *childishness* and *childish actions* were observed by:

Sir William Gowers.	Textbook on Nervous Diseases.
M. Bernhardt.	On Brain Tumours.
Henri Baruk.	Op. cit.
Dupres and Devaux.	Nouvelle Iconographie de la Salpétrière, 1901.
Soulaard.	Le puérelism mentale, Paris, 1904.
P. Courbon.	L'Encéphale, 1909.

Bouchard, Brissaud, Souques, Castan, Lejonne.

P. SCHUSTER (*Psychische Störungen bei Hirn Tumoren*, 1902) found irascibility a symptom in frontal tumours; but he included any and every case he could find in medical literature, even alcoholics and epileptics, in whom irascibility is a common symptom, and therefore not diagnostic of lesions of the frontal lobes.

EXAMPLES OF SURGICAL TREATMENT

BARTON and GAYTON (*British Medical Journal*, 1891): A woman, age 39, married, no family. There was a history of a blow on the head received whilst running upstairs, when she knocked her head against the top of the doorway. This spot, which was the seat of very great pain and headache, was selected for the operation, namely, one inch to the right of the middle line, and one inch behind the coronal suture. Patient had exalted ideas of wealth, delusions as to possessing carriages and horses, etc. There were no convulsions previous to the operation, but there were two afterwards. A fortnight later she began to improve, and from that time made a steady recovery. The delusions and headache were both cured. Before the operation she wrote badly and incoherently; after it her handwriting improved, and she wrote a reasonable letter. She was discharged.

T. Claye-Shaw (*British Medical Journal*, 1891): A man, age 36, a packer at the Army and Navy Stores, had, when admitted, grandiose delusions, and was impaired in both gait and speech. He was trephined by Mr. Harrison Cripps. The operation was carried out on the right side of the head, about the middle of the post-central convolution. There was considerable bulging of the tissues beneath the opening, indicating pressure. A considerable amount of fluid was drained away. Mental improvement followed. Patient became coherent, and had no delusions. He died suddenly in convulsions.

T. Claye Shaw (*Ibidem*, 1891): Another similar case.

H. S. Soutar (*British Medical Journal*, 1925): A woman, age 38, unstable mentally, acting with excitable levity in *abnormally high spirits*. Had a frontal tumour. Recovered after operation.

After all this evidence there can be no doubt as to euphoria and exaltation being symptoms of lesion of the frontal lobes, in contrast to the symptoms of mental depression and feeling of inferiority in lesion of the parietal lobes. But, if this is so, localisation of mental functions must be admitted, contrary to the opinion just now prevailing, and insanity should be studied from that point of view.

Frontal Lobes and Moral Degeneracy

The frontal brain is the seat of self-consciousness, a characteristic of the human being. By the growth of self-consciousness, and by means of introspection, understanding of social and moral law has been acquired, and inhibition developed. *The frontal lobes act as centres for inhibition;* that is to say, they enable us to exercise control over our feelings and impulses.

Plate XL

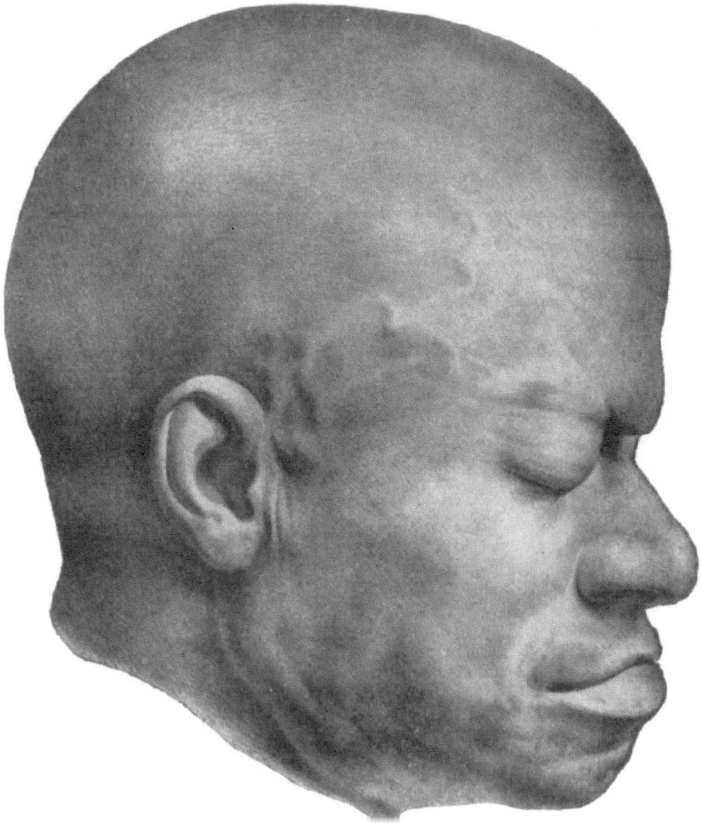

CAST OF HEAD OF A NEGRO, EUSTACHE OF ST. DOMINGO, RENOWNED FOR HIS BENEVOLENCE AND MORAL CHARACTER

Compare shape of head with that of Pope Alexander VI (*see page* 233)

Note.—*Plate* XXXIX *is printed on p. 221.*

In injury or disease of the frontal lobes, the intellect becomes affected, at least some element of it; but more manifest is the loss of inhibition over the natural dispositions. Consequently, these are manifested, not infrequently, in a much exaggerated manner. We see, thus, a creature given over to the satisfaction of his lower desires; a fact which accounts for the inaccurate statement, so often made, that frontal lesions may be accompanied by almost any symptom: irascibility, depression, etc. But these manifestations are not the symptoms; the only pathognomonic symptom is the loss of control over the natural tendencies.

The more developed the frontal lobes are, the more they overbalance the rest of the brain; consequently, the greater the tendency to subordinate the instincts of self-preservation, and the egoistic feelings, to the intellect, the greater the check on the animal propensities; the more deliberation, and the more moral the man. If this inhibition becomes weakened, or totally lost, then we see the disordered predominance of the instincts and impulses. These, being out of control, may lead the passionate man to immoral actions and the man with strong anti-social impulses to criminal deeds. This is the view, also, put forward and maintained by eminent Italian physiologists, notably POLIMANTI.

From this, one might wrongly conclude that the development of the moral sense is in proportion to the development of the intellect. But this is not so; for, as everyone knows, *there are moral idiots, as well as intellectual idiots*—men born with fair intellect, but with an entire absence of the higher moral sentiments, entirely destitute of moral feeling. They are as insensible to the moral relations of life—as deficient, in this regard, as is a colour-blind person to certain colours, or as one without ear for music is to the finest harmonies of sound. If caught in an immoral or criminal act, they show no repentance. They may perhaps feel and dread the material consequences of crime, but *they are deficient in the feeling of moral guilt.* They are not lacking in intelligence; their intellect is merely put to bad use.

Still, I agree with those who hold that *there are no definite centres in the brain for the manifestation of the moral sentiments.* But there are centres for adaptation and self-control, and that is what morality amounts to. These centres appear to be in the posterior part of the frontal lobes, which seem to act as a check to all the other centres. The actual locality is of no consequence, at present; so long as it is recognised that the moral sentiments may be lost in lesions of some portion of the brain. If a blow on the head can cause such circumscribed mental changes that only the *morality* of the man deteriorates, while he remains in all other respects unchanged, it shows that morality or immorality—that is, the tendency to one or the other—depends on brain conditions. And, if this be admitted, then we are also justified in assuming that the moral tendencies are subject to the laws of heredity; though *environmental influences and education will always discount, to a large extent, the innate disposition.*

The so-called moral sense is, of course, highly complex. Originating in the social sentiments, it is largely guided by the approbation of our fellow-men, ruled by reason, self-interest, religious feeling, and experience of the more remote consequences of our actions. But, in course of evolution, it has become part of the mental organisation, varying in degree in different people and dependent no longer so much on the approbation of others, as on the approbation of self; in other words, it has become—conscience. That it is not the product of a purely reflective faculty, is perceptible in children, from the earliest age. Some have it strongly, without teaching or example; others have it sparingly, and need the most assiduous care to develop it.

The larger the anterior lobes, in proportion to the rest of the brain, the more refined will be the expression of the emotions, and even of the passions of man; and the greater control will he be able to exert over them. Let the frontal lobes be arrested in development, as in idiocy, or affected by disease, and man descends to the animal stage. As the deficiency of the frontal lobes, in microcephalic brains, is not usually accompanied by a corresponding deficiency of the rest of the brain, the instincts in the mentally deficient, as in animals, are manifested more coarsely and vigorously from lack of any control by the intellect. All the propensities and emotions are present, except the higher emotions—the ethical, aesthetical, and spiritual—which belong to the frontal lobes, as we shall show. True, their emotions are not profound. A trivial event will make them laugh or cry, and it is easy to hurt their feelings with a slight offence; on the other hand, the death of a dear relative is very soon forgotten, while the stronger passions do not occur with that force and persistency common to normal man. The higher faculties that belong to the frontal lobes are, as I have said, absent. There is, for example, no idea of right and wrong. The higher idiots, certainly, experience a feeling of remorse, on offending the sympathies of those whom they love; but it seems, also, that even some dogs know when they have done wrong, and hide themselves from their master.

Ethical, aesthetical, and religious sentiments are formed, in the process of intellectual development. There are no centres for them in the brain; yet, in destructive lesions of the frontal lobes, owing to the reduction of the intellect, the altruistic sentiments (sympathy, kindness, charity) are frequently lost; the aesthetic sensibility, too, disappears, reducing the refined individual to a filthy and animal state, as seen in dementia. At first, there is impulsiveness, and incoherence of conduct; later, loss of initiative, and of volition in general (aboulia).

Every physician knows of the classical "Crowbar Case", recorded by Dr. HARLOW. It is so typical that it cannot be too often quoted. But it has been misrepresented in many of our textbooks, as showing that loss of brain substance may occur without any mental change; simply because the moral sentiments are not supposed to be dependent on brain matter. In his work on *The Functions of the Brain*, 1876, Sir DAVID FERRIER referred to the case of illustrating the fact that disease or injury to the frontal region in one hemisphere, is not followed by any appreciable mental symptoms. However, in his later work, *The Localisation of Cerebral Diseases*, 1878, he furnished a detailed account of it, proving the contrary. Nevertheless, in Kirkes' *Handbook of Physiology*, sixteenth edition, 1900, the crowbar case was still misrepresented, it being said that "no noteworthy symptoms were observed" in the patient "during the rest of his life"; indeed, he "returned to his work as overseer to the mine". This is not true. However, in answer to my protest, in later editions the case was left out altogether.

Another author falsely quoted the case as showing that the patient "lost nothing of mental power, of sagacity, and was entirely clear in all his mental processes".

The following is the actual history:

"While Phineas P. Gage, age 25, was engaged tamping a blasting charge in a rock, with a pointed iron bar 3 feet 7 inches in length, 1¼ inch in diameter, and weighing 13¼ pounds, the charge suddenly exploded. The iron bar, propelled with its pointed end first, entered at the left angle of the patient's jaw, and passed clean *through the top of his head near the sagittal suture in the frontal region*, and was picked up at some distance covered with blood and brains. The patient was for the moment stunned, but within an hour after the accident he was able to walk up a long flight of stairs, and give the surgeon an intelligible account of the injury he had sustained. His life was naturally for a long time despaired of, but he ultimately recovered, and lived 12½ years afterwards." This is what Dr. Harlow says of his mental condition during that period: "His contractors, who regarded him as the most efficient and capable foreman in their employ previous to his injury, considered the change in his mind so marked that they would not give him his place again. *The equilibrium or balance, so to speak, between the intellectual faculties and animal propensities, seems to have been destroyed.* He is fitful, irreverent, indulging at times in the grossest profanity (which was previously not his custom); manifesting but little deference for his fellows; impatient of restraint or advice when it conflicts with his desires; at times pertinaciously obstinate, yet capricious and vacillating; devising many plans of future operation, which are no sooner arranged than they are abandoned in turn for others appearing more feasible. *A child in his intellectual capacity and manifestations, he has the criminal passions of a strong man.* Previous to his injury, though untrained in the schools, he possessed a well-balanced mind, and was looked upon by those who knew him as a shrewd, smart business man, very energetic, and persistent in executing all his plans of operation. In this regard his mind was radically changed; so decidedly that his friends and acquaintances said he was 'no longer Gage'."

Gage became "very childish". He died 12½ years after the accident in epileptic convulsions. The base of the frontal bone was found fractured.

Case of Frontal Injury, Followed by Moral Insanity

Sir ROBERT ARMSTRONG-JONES (*Archives of Neurology*, 1907): X. Y., age 26, was admitted to Claybury Asylum from prison. The family history was singularly free from insanity and drink.

The patient was in good health and condition, and the organs apparently normal; traumatism being the assigned cause of insanity, patient having fallen forty feet from a lift, and fractured his skull in the pre-frontal region. The forehead showed a linear scar, six centimetres long, with obvious depression of the right frontal bone. Patient was unconscious for several days after the accident, and there was some loss of brain substance. Six months later some portions of dead bone were removed at St. Bartholomew's Hospital, and after two or three years of medical treatment he was pensioned as unfit for further work in Woolwich Arsenal. Before the accident, patient was bright, energetic, honest, and trustworthy; a life-abstainer, and much respected. After the accident there was complete metamorphosis; *his career became a record of moral obliquity and perversion.* He was idle, irritable, threatening, and violent; he was three times convicted of indecent behaviour, the last time he was ordered to be detained during His Majesty's pleasure, and after being in prison a month was removed to Claybury.

F. L. Goltz, although an opponent of the localisation theory, was a very accurate observer. He admitted that when the frontal lobes are destroyed, *the inhibitory power over the emotions and propensities is lost*; and such an animal changes its character for worse. His dogs, that were very docile and good-tempered, became, after removal of the frontal part of their brain, easily excited, irascible, made much noise, and were constantly disposed to fighting. In fact, it seems Goltz produced in his dogs symptoms similar to *mania* in man (*Die Verrichtungen des Grosshirns*, Bonn, 1881).

Jacques Loeb found the same as Goltz.

Bianchi (op. cit.) noted the absence of the moral sentiments, after destruction of the frontal lobes. He said: "Lesions of the frontal lobes do damage to the personality, and alter the individual character. That is the constant finding. *Not only animals operated upon, but also many men who suffer from extensive lesions of the frontal lobes, exhibit a profound alteration of character.* The actions of those who have suffered damage to the frontal lobes are impulsive in character; whilst the actions of healthy, well-developed men are deliberate, and based on experience, which, again, is bound up with representations and imagination. The defect that is most outstanding after mutilation of the frontal lobes, consists in the *entire absence of the higher sentiments*, whilst the primitive emotions remain sometimes even intensified, but not adapted for the struggle for existence in which these now inferior animals succumb. Bianchi also noticed that his mutilated animals had "no feeling for others", and observed that "a similar condition exists in human beings who have suffered severe injury to both frontal lobes, and in those whose frontal brains are imperfectly developed".

FLECHSIG (*Die Lokalisation der geistigen Vorgänge*, 1896) also observed "loss of ethical and aesthetical judgment" in lesions of the frontal lobes. He said: "The result of the action of physical impulses upon the cortex is a struggle between sensory impulses and reason. As soon as the power of the intellect is paralysed, the impulses are deprived of mental control, and passion reigns unbridled." He found in lesions of the frontal association centres that patients "*could not distinguish truth from untruth*, imagined events from experienced events, possible things from impossible. Ethical and aesthetical judgment diminished, prudence in the manifestation of the propensities was lost, self-control was gone. Finally, idiocy resulted with loss of personal identity".

CAMPBELL (*Journal of Mental Science*, 1904) declared—on histological evidence supplied by LEONORE WELT, and emphasised by v. MONAKOW—that "destruction of what one may call the middle part of the frontal lobe gives rise to various disturbances of the moral faculty."

WILLIAM BROWNING (*Medical Record*, 1921), after an analysis of *eleven cases* of cranial traumata, followed by a serious deterioration of moral conduct without intellectual weakening, placed the "moral centre", without hesitation, in the right frontal lobe.

L. B. BARKER, Professor of Anatomy and Pathology in Johns Hopkins University, said: "When the intellectual centres are paralysed, there often results most marked disorganisation of the mental processes, and *most serious alterations in the character* of the individual. The struggle between the lower instincts and the ethical feelings may cease, and instead of a rational man, we see a creature given over entirely to the satisfaction of his lower desires."

L. Canali (*Bulletin de la Société de Médicine Mentale*, 1881) recorded a case of brain lesion of the posterior end of the superior frontal convolution, followed by *moral insanity.*

W. C. Sullivan, formerly Superintendent of Broadmoor Criminal Lunatic Asylum, described several cases of *frontal brain tumour* in prisoners, and thought that their offences were due to loss of control over the lower instincts. Altogether, he found 4 per cent. of the total mortality of prisoners was due to brain tumour, a rather high proportion when it is borne in mind that cases of this disease, with distinct mental impairment, would not be likely to be sent to prison; or, if sent, would not be retained (*Lancet*, 1911).

Cases of Frontal Tumour with Loss of Moral Sense

F. X. Dercum (*Journal of Nervous and Mental Disease*, 1908): D. P., age 50, clergyman; family history and previous history good. *He used to be very conscientious, but now takes everything as a joke.* He has lost all sense of time, and can never keep an appointment. Gradually *he deteriorated morally.* Post-mortem, an enormous sarcomatous tumour was found involving both frontal lobes.

Rossolimo (*Deutsche Zeitschr. f. Nervenheilkunde*, 1895) had a patient suffering from *moral insanity*, in whom he found, post-mortem, a tumour at the top of the first and second right frontal convolutions.

Erich Feuchtwanger, in his book on *Stirntumoren*, Berlin, 1922, gave a case of burglary (No. 26), and another of fraud (No. 27), in which he found post-mortem frontal tumours.

The following is a case of frontal tumour, which caused moral degradation, and when removed by surgical operation, resulted in complete recovery of the patient:

PLATE XLI

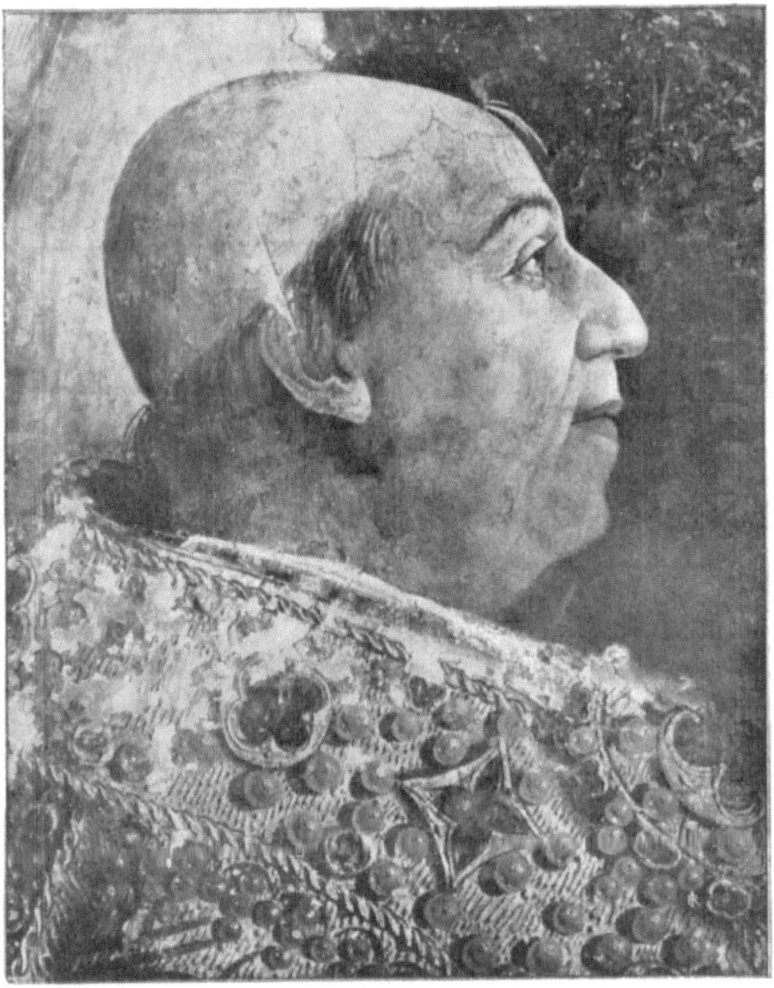

POPE ALEXANDER VI

Recorded to have been highly immoral

Compare shape of head with that of Eustache, Plate XL

Plate XLII

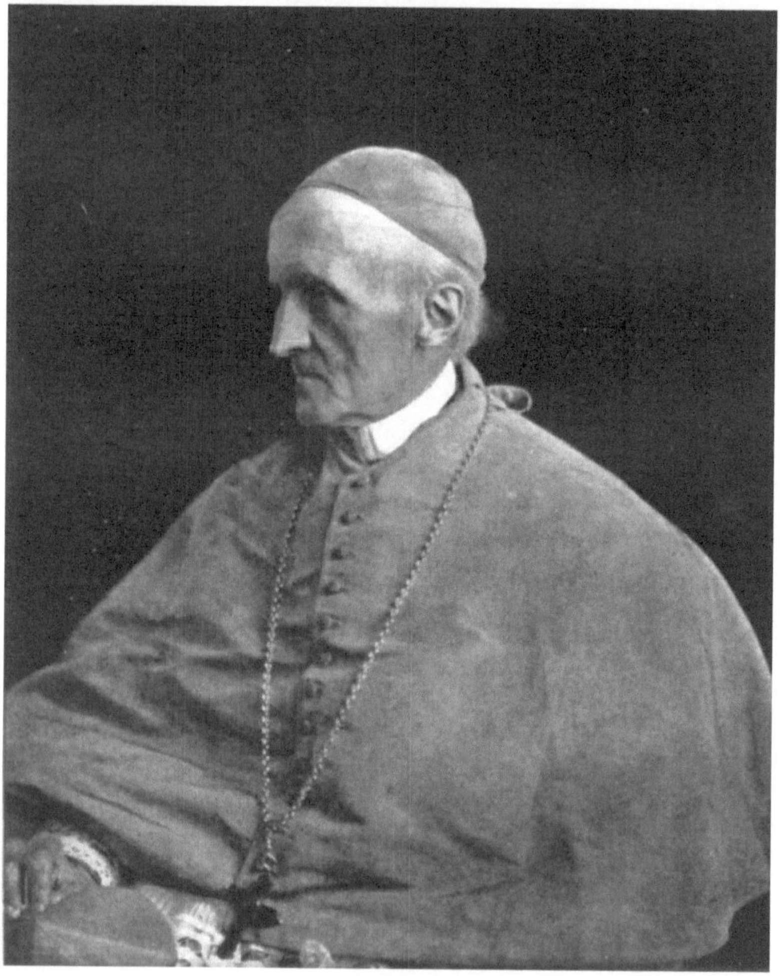

CARDINAL MANNING
Fine forehead. Mental temperament (*see page* 271)

Plate XLIII

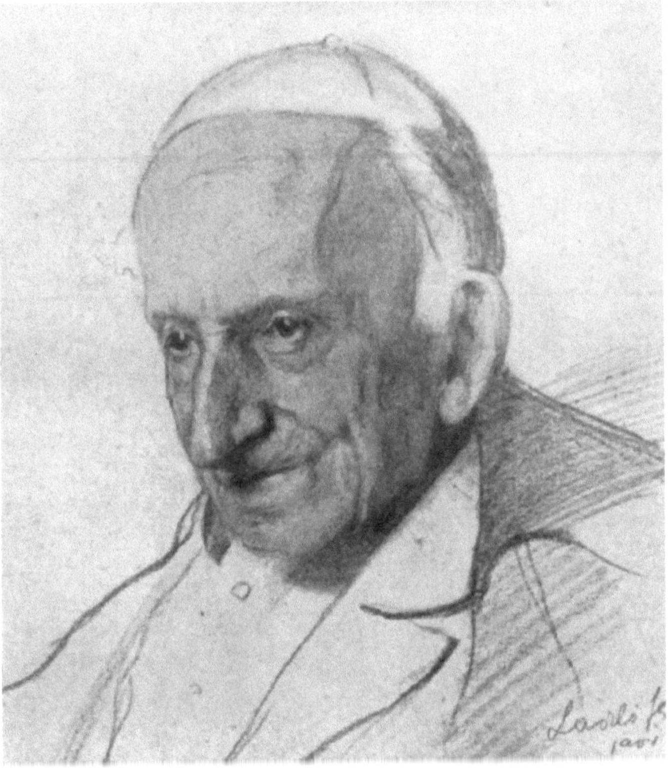

POPE LEO XIII

FRANCESCO DURANTE (*Supplem. al Policlinico*, 1896) recorded the case of a woman "previously shown at a Congress held in Perugia, suffering from loss of memory for words and things, religious perversions, *altered moral sense*, etc. Upon operating, a fibrous adherent body was found and removed. The patient changed, as if by magic, and speedily recovered her intellectual and moral faculties, and left the hospital sound."

Professor Durante has observed other cases of frontal tumour, in which "the intellectual disturbances had assumed the character of *moral insanity*.

Moral changes in lesions of the frontal lobes were observed also by the following:

H. Schüle.	Sektionsergebnisse b. Geisteskranken, 1874. *After head injury in the frontal region.*
Leonore Welt.	Archiv. f. Klinische Medizin, 1888.
Raymond.	Leçons Cliniques, Paris, 1892.
Obici.	Il Policlinico, 1895.
Bruns.	Geschwülste d. Nervensystems, Berlin, 1897.
Pierre Marie.	Revue Neurologique, 1894.
Byrom Bramwell.	Brain, 1899.
H. Oppenheim.	Geschwülste des Gehirns, 1902.
John B. Chapin.	American Journal of Insanity, 1862. *Case of tumour at vertex of brain.*
Vögelin.	Allg. Zeitschrift f. Psychiatrie, 1898. *Frontal tumour.*
Gianelli.	Policlinico, 1897. *Two cases of frontal tumour.*
E. Brown.	Alienist and Neurologist, 1883. *After frontal head injury.*

Dr. RICHARD EAGER (*Journal of Mental Science*, 1920) is opposed to this theory. He said: "From the cases that have passed through my hands, there seems to be no uniformity in the psychic symptoms that may follow frontal injuries, and the tendency that there has been, in the past, to consider, as a special characteristic of injuries in this region, the likelihood of the moral character of the individual to suffer most, is not supported." Dr. Eager appears to me to have overlooked the fact mentioned by me in earlier chapters, that this region at the top of the head, at the posterior border of the frontal lobes, is often covered for an inch or two by the anterior upper extremity of the parietal bones; for he gives two cases of moral degeneracy subsequent to a frontal injury, but puts them under lesions of the parietal region.

The first of these cases was that of a boy age 19, well educated, and hitherto of exemplary character. After some "irritability", which subsided, the patient showed a type of "pseudologia phantastica". He became a notorious liar, and full of deceit in every conceivable way. He had, also, tendencies to kleptomania.

The other case is that of a soldier who had received an injury, again vaguely described as "a shell wound in the right parietal region". This man, formerly well behaved, had become "most unreliable, and had three court-martials, and practically lived in detention". "No punishment seemed to make the slightest impression on him, and he had taken to drink and other bad habits, which were previously quite foreign to his nature."

Considering how rare it is that character changes are observed at all by physicians and surgeons, the evidence I have given must be regarded as sufficient to warrant a systematic investigation. It must be remembered (as I have already explained) that the hospital is not the best place in which to observe loss of special abilities or moral changes. Neither abilities nor conduct can be judged while the patient is still in bed. We must wait until he attempts to return to active life and his profession. I have seen a number of men with head injuries, who were discharged from hospitals as sound, but proved failures in their vocations; and several of them manifested marked criminal tendencies.

If experimental physiology can be relied upon, then, of course, the evidence produced in this chapter is absolutely valueless. For, if we look at the later maps of the motor field of the brain, when the groups of muscles had been described in greater detail, we find, *at the top of the frontal brain, the centres for movements of the anus, vagina,* and other structures, which no doubt have to perform necessary functions; but it is difficult to believe that the highest development of the frontal lobes, which gives such a dome-like appearance to the living head (see illustrations) should have for its function that of assisting defaecation and coitus.

CHAPTER XII

CRANIO-CEREBRAL RELATIONS

Can we estimate the size and shape of the brain from the outline of the skull? Certainly we can, and this is the view of nearly all the anatomists, from the ancient time of GALEN, to BLUMENBACH, MAGENDIE, GRATIOLET, CUVIER, BROCA, MANOUVRIER, WELCKER, VIRCHOW, ZUCKERKANDL, ECKER, OBERNIER, SIR CHAS. BELL, S. G. MORTON, and modern anatomists.

There can be not the slightest doubt that the skull represents, for all practical purposes, a true measure of the dimensions of the growth of that organ. Wrong conclusions had been drawn from the appearance of the brain when removed from the skull. Then, of course, being no longer supported on all sides, it sinks down and flattens out; though it has filled the cranial cavity completely during life.

Those who deny that the skull and brain conform in outline would have us believe that the brain obeys the inert resistance of the cranium because the latter is the harder, in spite of evidence afforded to the contrary, in the case of hydrocephalic subjects. They forget that the skull is a living substance, and that there is a continual process going on of absorption, nutrition, decomposition, and new formation of osseous molecules. They forget, also, that the continual action of nature in nutrition changes and modifies the hardest of substances as easily as the softest parts, through the successive apposition of nutritive elements and the reabsorption of those that have remained a long while in the system. They should remember, moreover, that the skull cavity is so closely filled by the brain that any development of it must exert pressure on its own substance—with serious consequences—unless that part of the skull becomes elevated. Does not the shell of the snail, and the shield of the tortoise, expand with the increase of the animal? Why? Because the hard covering is made for the protection of the animal, and not the animal for the covering. Likewise the brain is not made for the skull, but the osseous envelope is certainly made to protect the brain. The brain being an object more essential to the end of nature than the skull, quite obviously, the latter should yield to the development of the former, and everything tends to prove that it does.

It is a general physiological fact that the hard parts of the body are adapted to the size and form of the soft ones they enclose. In consumption, if one side of the lungs alone be affected, the ribs of that side sink down. If the eye be extirpated, the orbit becomes smaller; and if, on the contrary, it becomes carcinomatous, the orbit enlarges, as the eyeball increases in size. Precisely so does the skull follow the brain, in its size and general configuration.

Skulls vary in thickness; but since nature, in forming the bony frame of healthy people, has a uniform mode of working, a healthy man may be judged to have a thick skull, if the other bones of the body are also strong and thick. On the other hand, we may infer from thin bones of the limbs a comparative thinness of skull under normal conditions.

It seems strange that such a simple problem—whether the skull fits the brain—should not have been settled long ago. The fact is, few trouble their heads about it, otherwise it would be solved every day, in any dissecting-room. I have carefully observed many dissections, seen the skull sawn through, and the brain exposed; and *I have never failed to observe that, when the skull-cap was lifted off, the brain showed exactly the same elevations and depressions as did the skull.* It is sufficient to say that brain shape does, in the main, undoubtedly determine skull shape in human beings, at least in normal cases. Any deviation between the two skull plates, when it exists, amounts, usually, only to *one-tenth or two-tenths of an inch,* except at the frontal sinus and the occipital protuberance; whereas the differences in the development of particular regions of the head amount to entire inches. Even if single convolutions do not always impress themselves perceptibly on the outer surface of the skull, groups of convolutions do modify the shape of the cranium; indeed, *there are no two skulls alike,* as little as there are two faces alike.

Every child is born with a tendency to that form of brain which it afterwards assumes. To allow of this, the brain of the foetus is not surrounded by any osseous substance, but by a transparent, cartilaginous membrane, which becomes osseous simply for the protection of the brain. The forehead, which, in a newly born infant, is perpendicular, or flattened backward, begins to protrude as soon as its life ceases to be purely vegetative, passed between sleeping and feeding, and it begins to take notice of the external world. As the child observes, and begins to reason, the small, narrow, short forehead of the early months dilates in all directions, and especially forward; the frontal bone increases in convexity with the rapidly growing frontal lobes of the brain, and in relation to the extensive knowledge he now acquires. Later on, these frontal parts get more balanced with the rest of the brain, and the little prodigy resumes his place among ordinary folk.

The inferior part of the occipital bone also undergoes marked changes. In the new-born infant it is very slightly developed, as compared with the rest of the brain. The cranium is contracted in this region, resembling a truncated cone. The external prominences, corresponding to the occipital fossae, are small, flat, and almost imperceptible. The two mastoid processes are still very near each other. But mark the difference in the boy arrived at puberty. The occipital fossae are distinctly observable externally by their protuberances. The mastoid processes are much further separated. The posterior base is far larger. Finally, in more mature age, the prominences corresponding to the occipital fossae are much larger still, so that the base of the cranium, taken from one temporal bone to the other, equals almost its diameter.

The enlargement I have just described in the case of these two situations takes place, in like manner, when other cerebral parts get more developed; and, considering the thinness of the cranium, one can recognise from it, with certainty, the shape of the brain.

Brain growth is the determining factor, and the skull grows upon, and accommodates itself to, the brain—whether the latter be large or small. Surgeons who have removed strips of bone from the skulls of microcephalic idiots, with the idea of affording more space and freedom for the growth of the brain, have evidently forgotten this fact; hence their failure.

Idiots are such because of arrested brain growth, generally intra-uterine; and not, as at one time many surgeons believed, because of arrested skull growth. The false assumption that, in mentally deficient children, the skull closes prematurely and presses upon the brain, has led to the futile operation described. A microcephalic brain is not a more or less normal brain, only very small in size—the idiocy resulting from the smallness of the parts present; but it is always an abnormal and undeveloped, and, in a great many instances, a diseased brain. Large areas of it may never be developed, and the cells that are present are small and comparatively few in number. If a strip of bone be removed from the skull, new normal brain cells will not be produced; *parts that are entirely absent cannot be created, and powers that do not exist cannot be called into being.* The reported improvement after this operation is not due to the surgical procedure. Many cases have been reported at too early a date, and the improvement has not continued. When it has done so, it has more likely been due to proper instruction and care, and not to the operation. *It is different, however, in cases of feeble-mindedness where there is a history of head-injury.* In these there may be pressure of a fragment of bone, or extravasated blood on the brain, and trephining called for.

After the period of maturity, the cranium thickens by degrees in the following manner. The bones of the cranium are composed of two solid osseous layers, or laminae, representing the external and internal surfaces, respectively; the space between these two laminae is filled with a cellular substance, or diploe. This substance is, however, not of a uniform thickness throughout, so that the two tables are more separated from each other at some places than at others. Thus, although the internal surface of the cranium is exactly moulded on the surface of the brain—from the moment when the cranium has acquired a certain thickness, it cannot be asserted, without qualification, that its external surface exactly represents the convolutions of the brain. The two tables of the cranium are no longer parallel in their whole circumference. Now, does this want of parallelism between the two tables of the skull, in men whose brain has reached or passed maturity, really prevent one from arriving at a conclusion as to the development of the brain beneath? Such lack of parallelism between the two tables of the cranium rarely occurs at the top, nor in the squamous area at the sides; and those are, in many respects, the most important regions. Therefore, a deviation of about one-tenth or two-tenths of an inch, to which I have alluded, cannot be of great significance, in view of the fact that differences in the development of particular regions of the head amount, commonly, to entire inches.

As regards the skulls of the insane, the cranium, when the mental derangement has been of short duration, may be enlarged in a particular segment; but often does not offer the least trace of diseased alteration. When, however, the brain disease has been chronic, a wasting may take place, the whole brain may shrink; and the bones may thicken, become more dense, compact, and heavier, approaching somewhat the texture of ivory. Many idiots, too, when the idiocy is not due to hydrocephalus, have a very thick cranium.

That the skull-bones have the power to adapt themselves to abnormal conditions has been shown by A. B. Drousik (*On the Causes influencing the Shape of the Skull*, St. Petersburg, 1883), who stated, as the result of his experiments on animals, firstly, that the skull-bones increase in thickness, in proportion to the diminution of pressure (reduced activity) on the part of the brain, from the inner surface; secondly, that an abnormal development of the brain, as well as any changes in its form, influences the configuration of the skull and, indirectly, of the face.

F. A. Lange and J. Engel held that the shape of the cranium depends on the *traction* certain muscles (the masticatory muscles in front and the neck muscles at the back) exert on the head. In answer to this objection, let me point out (1) that the muscles are softer than the cranium; (2) that notwithstanding the muscles, the head increases in size; and (3) that the base of the brain is a solid structure, which does not change much, and is harder for the protection of the more vital organs at the base of the brain—not like the vault of the skull, where the almost immovable occipito-frontalis muscle is attached. If the muscles really determined the form of the skull, they ought, obviously, to act in the direction of their insertions; and the protuberances of the occiput and sides of the head ought, then, to be directed downwards; not backwards, and to the sides. There ought, also, to be some proportion between the size of these protuberances and the strength of the muscles inserted between them; but it often happens that large protuberances correspond to weak muscles, and vice versa.

The brain is frequently described as lying upon a water-bed, or as swimming in the *cerebro-spinal fluid.* The only portions which are really separated from the skull are the medulla oblongata and the pons Varolii, structures containing the centres controlling the action of the circulatory and respiratory organs, and other vital functions, and may therefore be regarded as the most vital parts of the central nervous system, which need special protection. Otherwise the amount of fluid in the subdural space is only enough to prevent friction during the movements of the brain.

The difficulty, with reference to the *frontal sinus,* has also been much exaggerated. In children, one may ignore it altogether. The sinus does not generally appear before the age of twelve. After puberty it is generally present, and increases with age. In women, the frontal sinus is smaller than in men; and only slight allowances need be made.

In men, the bodily constitution will tell us what sized sinus to expect. Where all the bones are large, the sinus may be expected to be large, though not necessarily so. In old age, chronic idiocy, and dementia, it may be of abnormal size. Finally, the frontal sinus, even when excessively developed, affects only the centre part of the lowest segment of the frontal lobes of the brain, and does not affect the width of that part of the forehead or its length from the ear forward.

All these difficulties exist only for those who look for protuberances on the head; they do not affect the scientific man, who looks, first, at the general configuration of the head; then at the development of the different bones which make up the skull, in order to judge of the size of the various lobes of the brain underneath; and who has a scientific system of measurement, not of one direction only, but including the length, breadth, width, and height of each region.

If the brain and skull do not agree in conformation, one may well ask what is the good of anthropometry, craniology, anthropology, and all the other studies that are based on measurements of heads.

It is surprising how many men of high reputation as scientists and physiologists used to speak of "bumps" and called it "quackery and deceit" to determine the size and shape of the brain by the size and shape of the skull. One well-known University professor declared that "it would be just as possible for a safe-maker to examine the knob or handle of a safe, and then profess to be able to tell what amount of wealth was contained in the safe in its various drawers and compartments". Another, a distinguished professor of physiology, said: "It is just as reasonable to determine a person's digestive capacity by looking at his waistcoat, as it is to pretend to know the shape of the brain by looking at the skull." It would have been easy to verify this; but there are none so blind as those who do not want to see.

Nowadays, it is not the teachers in medical colleges, but the lecturers on psychology who tell us that "the skull does not correspond to the brain formation". Why they should go out of their way to spread such a fable, when, in all likelihood, they have never seen a head dissected, is difficult to understand. I could give several examples from recent books on psychology, but one illustration will suffice. Thus F. W. WESTAWAY has given us a learned treatise on *Scientific Method*, in which he explains that "The great characteristic of scientific method is verification at every stage . . . for we cannot completely rid ourselves of the old habit of hastily taking up opinions which we have not properly examined". Quite true; but unfortunately the author has not followed the instruction he gives to others, and cites as an "instance of the manner in which numerous coincidences may mislead the unscientific mind" when the assumption is made "that the outside of the skull is so finely and accurately modelled to the surface of the brain that it is an exact copy of that surface, *an assumption which has been absolutely disproved*".

The pity is that with such authoritative opinions, pronounced as they sometimes are from professorial chairs, the error gets widespread, and the knowledge which could be gained from the observation of the size and shape of the head is absolutely neglected. Since these critics are not likely to accept my own observations made in dissecting-rooms, I am quoting here the observations of the greatest British anatomists, to settle the matter for all times.

Sir GEORGE M. HUMPHRY, Professor of Anatomy, Cambridge University, said: "The skull is moulded upon the brain, and grows in accordance with it. The size and general shape of the brain may be estimated with tolerable accuracy by the size and general shape of the skull. The frontal sinuses and the projecting ridges—the inequalities on the surface of the skull, which have no correspondence in the interior, do not amount to much, and do not affect the principle that the skull is moulded upon and fitted to the brain; and that its exterior does, as a general rule, convey pretty accurate information respecting the size and shape of that organ."

Sir WILLIAM TURNER, Professor of Anatomy in Edinburgh University, and a pioneer in cranio-cerebral topography, drew attention to the fact that in certain regions the outer surface of the skull possesses elevations and depressions which closely correspond to definite fissures and convolutions of the brain, and he added (*West Riding Lunatic Asylum Medical Reports*, Vol. III) that "single psychical functions, and probably all, are related to circumscribed centres of the cortex of the cerebrum".

Sir DAVID FERRIER, one of the greatest authorities on the brain, who also studied cranio-cerebral relations, made the following statements (*Harveian Oration*, 1902):

1. The brain fills the cranial cavity like a hand in a glove, and is closely appressed to the interior of the skull-cap.

2. Under normal conditions, the amount of cerebro-spinal fluid is so small as to be practically a negligible quantity.

3. As a general rule, it is not till about the fortieth year that the cranial sutures (except at the base) become ankylosed, and the process is not completed till much later in life.

4. So long as the intersutural fibrous tissue is present, the cranium may increase.

5. Increase of the brain pressure from within can delay the closure of the sutures.

Professor ALEXANDER MACALISTER, of Cambridge University, said: "The largest part of the skull is that which is at once the receptacle and the protector of the brain; a part which, when unmodified by external pressure, premature synostosis, or other adventitious conditions, owes its form to that of the cerebral hemispheres which it contains. . . . So far from the shape of the brain being seriously modified by the constraining influence of the surrounding embryonic skull, the form of the soft membranous brain case is previously moulded upon the brain within it, whose shape may, however, be to some extent a secondary agent in modifying its later growth. We have also learned that the cerebrum is not a single organ acting as a functional unit, but consists of parts, each of which has its specific province; that the increase in the number of cells in any area is correlated with an increase in the size and the complexity of pattern of the convolutions of that area; and that this, in turn, influences the shape of the enclosing shell of membrane, and subsequently of bone" (*British Association Meeting*, Edinburgh, 1892).

D. J. Cunningham, Professor of Anatomy, at the British Association Meeting, Glasgow, 1901, said: "The cranium is the outward expression of the contained brain, and the brain is the most characteristic organ of man; cranial peculiarities, therefore, must always, and should always, claim a leading place in the mind of the anthropologist. During the development of the brain, the cranium expands according to the demands made upon it by the growing brain. The initiative lies with the brain, and in normal conditions it is questionable if the envelope exercises more than a very subsidiary and limited influence upon the form assumed by the contents. The directions of growth are clearly defined by the sutural lines by which the cranial bones are knit together; but these are so arranged that they admit of the expansion of the cranial box in length, in breadth, and in height, and the freedom of growth in each of these different directions has, in all probability, been originally determined by the requirements of the several parts of the brain. *The cranial vault fits like a tight glove on the surface of the enclosed cerebrum.* The cortical elevations which rise on the surface are due to exuberant growth in localised areas. There cannot be a doubt that the process is intimately connected with the development of function in the districts concerned. We know that functions of different kinds are localised in different parts of the cortex, and *when we see an area on the cerebrum rise up in the form of an eminence we may reasonably conclude that the growth in the area concerned is the structural foundation of what will become later on a centre of functional activity of an acute kind.*" He recommended the study of skull peculiarities, brains seldom being available for investigation to any but medical men.

Professor SYMINGTON, of Belfast University, at the British Association Meeting, 1903, said: "It is the brain growth that determines the form of the cranium; and not the skull that moulds the brain into shape. There can be no doubt that, within certain limits, *the external form of the cranium serves as a reliable guide to the shape of the brain.* Indeed, various observers have drawn attention to the fact that in certain regions the outer surface of the skull possesses elevations and depressions which closely correspond to definite fissures and convolutions of the brain."

Sir ARTHUR KEITH (*Henderson Trust Lecture*, Edinburgh University, 1924) said: "The brain and its house, the skull, grow and expand together; the developing brain, as a whole, and also each of its individual departments, have the power to enlarge and modify its containing walls of bone according to needs. *The size and form of the skull do depend on the form and size of the brain;* and form and size of brain do depend on the organisation of the central nervous system."

Professor G. ELLIOT SMITH (*Henderson Trust Lecture*, Edinburgh University, 1923): "The brains of the primitive members of the human family, as well as of representatives of the existing races, reveal the fact that profound differences do occur between human brains; and that they are due in the main to the localised hypertrophy or the localised atrophy of definite regions, rather than of the brain as a whole. Moreover, it can now be demonstrated that *it is the growth of the brain which determines the size and form of the skull, and not vice versa.* If the cortex of the brain of an unborn foetus, or a cat, or a rabbit be destroyed by administering radium to the mother, the young will go on living after birth, although the brain ceases to grow; and, in such cases, it is found that the skull ceases to expand when the brain does. . . . These facts afford some corroboration that there is a definite localisation of function in the brain, that localised hypertrophies do occur; that the skull adapts itself to the form assumed by the brain. Therefore, it can be assumed that *the form and size of the brain case must have some relationship to the individual's aptitudes.*"

CHAPTER XIII

THE EXTERNAL SIGNS OF INTELLIGENCE

Practical Application of the Localisation Theories

If we never look at the outline of a living head, an *important aid to diagnosis in mental deficiency* is lost to us, apart from other practical uses. The number and post-mortem appearances of the microscopical brain cells, on which Insanity and Mental Deficiency textbooks lay great stress, will not help us with the diagnosis or treatment of *living* imbeciles and the mentally deranged. And, while the mental tests practised so extensively in our elementary schools are, undoubtedly, excellent, they would gain still more in value if, in addition, any exceptional shape of the head were taken notice of. For instance, a broad, high, and prominent frontal region, with flat posterior development, must have some significance, when compared, say, with a low, narrow, sloping forehead and large occiput. On the other hand, when a child's head is elongated and prominent, both front and back, having abnormal dimensions, it should arouse suspicion of an excess of cerebro-spinal fluid, that is to say, of actual or arrested hydrocephalus.

To judge of the development of a head, *imagine a vertical plane, midway between the two ears.* All the part which lies in front of that plane is—roughly speaking—concerned with the intellectual functions; all the part which lies behind that plane is concerned with the emotions and passions. But remember, even if the frontal lobes be large, this does not, necessarily, signify superiority of intellect, for the brain structure may be simple; or, if up to the average, it may never have been stocked with knowledge or experiences. Such a brain resembles an empty warehouse, in which no goods have been deposited.

The fore-brain reasons and knows; creates ideas; forms plans; evolves methods; analyses laws and principles; understands, comprehends, discriminates; exercises the elements of insight, perception, or discernment.

To judge of the size of the fore-brain we must look, first of all, at *the extent of its base*, from the opening of the ear to the outer corner of the eyebrow; a line which, on the average, measures two and a half inches. Below that measure is indicated poverty of intellect; above it, superior capacity.

Next, we must look at the *height of the plane*, from the opening of the ear to the top of the head; and notice, also, how much the head rises above the frontal eminences in the upper part of the forehead. For, sometimes—especially in men with a violent temperament—the temporal region may be highly developed so that the ears are fixed very low, which makes the head appear high, unless we observe the height of the head above the frontal eminences as well. I have seen murderers, while under remand, whose heads the Prison Governor had considered to resemble those of Bishops, until I called his attention to the fact that the head hardly rose above these protuberances. Looked at from the front, they had low heads; but from the side, they appeared to have high heads.

Lombroso and other craniologists have noticed large temporal lobes in violent criminals. This, as I have said, causes the ears to be rather low; but there is a definite measure. In mildly disposed persons the ear is almost at the level of the outer corner of the eye, so that the angle formed by a line drawn from the corner of the eye to the opening of the ear, and from the ear to the opening of the nose, is at most fifteen to twenty degrees. In the violent man, however, with large temporal lobes, this angle may measure as much as forty-five degrees.

Let me point out here, that *there is no distinctly criminal type of head.* A highly developed intellect may serve for the gratification of the instinctive desires. The typical criminal of the criminologists, in the past, was a man who, among other signs, had a very small frontal region, which, we know, indicates feeble-mindedness. Our prison population consists, largely, of weak-minded men and women. The clever criminal escapes, at least for a great length of time.

FLECHSIG claimed that the height of the forehead depended on the volume of the sensory sphere; and this in turn on the volume of the body. The height of the forehead, in his opinion, was not a direct index to mental ability. This comes from not looking at living heads. I have dealt in Chapter V with those craniologists who claim that a high forehead indicates healed-up hydrocephalus.

Next, we must look at the *vaulting of the frontal bones.* A sloping forehead will not contain as much fore-brain as a highly vaulted one. Never forget that you are looking at only one surface. *A receding forehead is quite compatible with marked intellectual power, if the breadth, height, and depth of the frontal lobes are good*

From this it will be seen that, in estimating the size of the frontal lobes, it is not a question of isolated depressions or elevations; but the development of their whole extent, which we must measure, actually, or by the eye.

Having measured the entire front region, we can then look at certain parts of it.

A forehead which is *prominent over the eyebrows* signifies a keen observer, practical talents, mechanical ability. Such a man, with the lower forehead large, takes more interest in facts than in arguments, deals with practical things in a practical way.

The *upper part of the forehead is prominent* (as measured from the opening of the ears across the frontal eminences) in the man of meditation and reflection; the man who wants to know the reason for everything. It is prominent in the scholar and in the philosopher (see illustrations).

A *very high forehead* is an indication of lofty ideals, vivid imagination, lofty sentiments, appreciation of the beautiful; it denotes a sympathetic nature. This type is aspiring, idealistic, and rises above material desires. The world's great poets, creators of fine arts, benefactors, reformers, and geniuses, have mostly had high foreheads (see illustrations). *But we must not forget that imagination is needed, not only by the poet and artist, but that it is, also, the handmaiden of science and needed by the statesman; indeed, by all men who can lay claim to the creative ability.* Look, for example, at Mussolini's head.

Remarkable foreheads may be seen amongst working-class men. Some, though they possess no special knowledge, are able to propound sound, practical views on the problems of life; while a great many others have studied for themselves politics, political economy, and even special science, in which they excel. Some may be animated by a strong curiosity to know; may be plodding and persevering; and gifted with concentration for one line of study, without being remarkable in anything else.

The expansion of the frontal lobes in men by intellectual training has been repeatedly demonstrated by actual measurements. An acquaintance of mine, a teacher, who took some measurements of London County Council schoolboys, some years ago, made some interesting observations.

He found: (1) that the most intellectual boys averaged half an inch more anterior than posterior brain, whereas the least intellectual boys possessed half an inch more posterior than frontal brain; (2) that younger but more intellectual boys had not only slightly larger heads, as shown by the circumference, than older but duller boys in the same class, but that the ratio between the anterior and posterior measurements in the former was much greater than in the latter; (3) that the anterior measurement of the brain, in boys passing up from Standard I to VII, increased at a greater rate than the posterior measurement in accordance with the increase of their intellectual capacity.

HERMANN WAGNER, inspired by his father RUDOLF WAGNER, in 1864, compared the mean proportion of the cortex in man and the orang. The occipital lobes proved larger in the orang than in man; while the frontal lobes were considerably smaller. He also weighed each lobe of the brain of Gauss, the mathematician, and of other eminent men, and compared it with the weight obtained from the brains of working-class men. The workmen had the smallest frontal lobes, but they had larger occipital lobes than the celebrated mathematician.

The important researches made in reference to ancient skulls by the ABBÉ FRÈRE, whose rich collection is in the Anthropological Museum at Paris, led him to the conclusion that the skulls of Europeans have increased in size since historic times; and that *the progress of civilisation seems to have resulted in raising the anterior, and flattening the occipital, part of the skull.*

PAUL BROCA examined the heads of 32 house-surgeons, who had successively resided at the Bicêtre during the years 1861–2, and compared the dimensions with those of the heads of 24 porters, attached to the various wards of the same hospital. This comparison resulted in the confirmation of the generally received opinion, that the anterior lobes are the instruments for the higher intellectual operations; and Broca considered that he had demonstrated that *the cultivation of the mind and intellectual work augment the size of the brain; and that such increase affects chiefly the anterior lobes* (*Revue Scientifique*, 1861–2).

J. B. M. PARCHAPPE also made measurements, and found that the frontal lobes in men of learning have much larger proportion than in the average man of the working classes.

LACASSAGNE and CLIQUET have examined by aid of the conformateur the heads of 190 doctors of medicine, 133 rudimentarily educated persons, 90 illiterate persons, and 91 prisoners (soldiers), with the following results. There was a considerable difference in size of head, in favour of the doctors; and this was especially marked in the frontal measurement. In the educated, the frontal region was more developed on the left side, and was altogether proportionately more developed than the occipital region, which in the case of the illiterate was the larger.

ALEXANDER MACALISTER, Professor of Anatomy, at the British Association Meeting, Edinburgh, 1892, declared that "increased growth of the frontal lobes is the physical accompaniment of intellectual activity".

SCHRÖDER VAN DER KOLK wrote: "That to all parts of the cerebral convolutions are not assigned exactly similar functions was long ago suspected. Further, that a finely arched forehead indicates, as a rule, high intellectual endowment was not unknown to the Greeks, as we may conclude from their delineations of Jupiter, Apollo, and so forth. The strongly prominent forehead as the prerogative of man came yet more definitely into view when Camper proposed the facial angle named after him, and pointed out its difference in Azteks, Negroes, and Europeans, in children likewise and in grown-up persons."

Sometimes the frontal part of the head looks small when compared with the size of the rest of the head, and yet there may be considerable intellectual power. In such cases it will generally be found, owing to vigorous emotions and instincts, that the intelligence receives more than ordinary stimulation. Some men are moved by strong ambition, or are more plodding and persevering; others know better how to make the best use of what little knowledge they possess. Besides, there are people who distinguish themselves in one special field of knowledge without being possessed of all-round intelligence.

If *the head is very broad* from ear to ear (when the diameter between the two ears is very big)—the result of well-developed temporal lobes—this is an indication of working capacity, force of character and energy, industry, executive ability, determination, reserve energy, and kindred elements. And this principle applies, equally, whether the head be a large or a small one. This breadth gives physical stamina, and is therefore fitted for aggressive work—for driving through obstacles. The bullet-shaped head is the fighting head. Broad temporal regions and big jaws often go together, indicating the man of fight and push. Compare, for instance, the head of a prize-fighter with that of a Catholic Bishop. Compare, also, the brain of a lion with that of a lamb.

According to Sir ARTHUR KEITH (*Henderson Trust Lecture*, 1924) men of the neolithic age—about 2000 B.C.—"were men with massive, strong faces, frowning and burly supra-orbital ridges, of great strength of body, and with peculiarly flattened occiputs. Their heads were said to be 'rounded', because it happened in most of them that *the width of the skull was* 80 *per cent. or more of its length.*"

Sir Arthur Keith's observation can be interpreted in accordance with the theories advanced in this book: that the heads of neolithic men were extraordinarily wide, because they had to fight for their existence; and they had the orbital region highly developed for the same reason; for they had to be observant, in order to escape destruction, though, no doubt, the prominent ridges were due partly to the size of their frontal sinuses (see illustrations).

Labourers, from the nature of their work and the greater

struggle for existence, call their animal impulses more into action, and hence require relatively larger temporal lobes than men of learning. That this is actually the fact was shown by Hermann Wagner—to whom I have already referred—whose measurements revealed that the size of the temporal lobes in an uneducated labourer was as 30 to 100, the latter figure representing the entire brain mass; while in men of learning it was as 25 to 100. On the other hand, the size of the frontal lobes in men of learning was as 40 to 100, while in a labourer it was only as 36 to 100. Wagner's observations, therefore, prove to us that the temporal lobes are not only larger in the labourer than in the man of learning, as 30 to 25, but that they are a great deal larger, because we must take into account that the frontal lobes are smaller, as 36 to 40, and thus, by exercising less control, impart greater power to the functions of the temporal lobes.

A large development of the temporal lobes indicates great strength of the animal passions and of the physiological and vital force of the constitution. If the breadth of the head is balanced by a proportionate development of the intellectual and moral region, the character will be strong, yet attractive. We must never estimate the strength of the animal dispositions by the size of the temporal lobes alone, but only in conjunction with the development of the rest of the brain—particularly the size of the entire frontal lobes, the intellectual and moral regions—which inhibit, or at least modify, the manifestation of the instincts originally intended for self-preservation.

The *narrow-headed* man (with small temporal lobes) is mild, easy-going, diplomatic; he prefers to gain his purpose by persuasion and tact rather than by despotic, destructive

Plate XLIV

ILLUSTRATIONS OF THE THREE PRINCIPAL TEMPERAMENTS

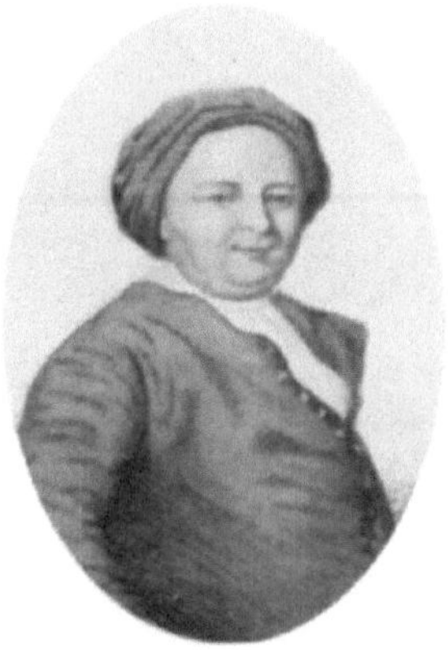

Vital Temperament

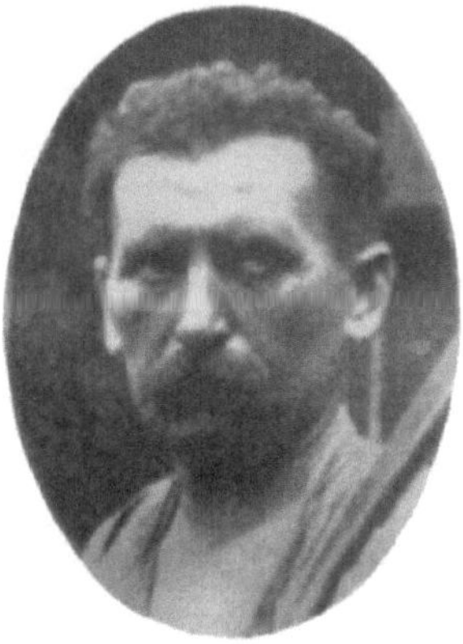

Motive Temperament

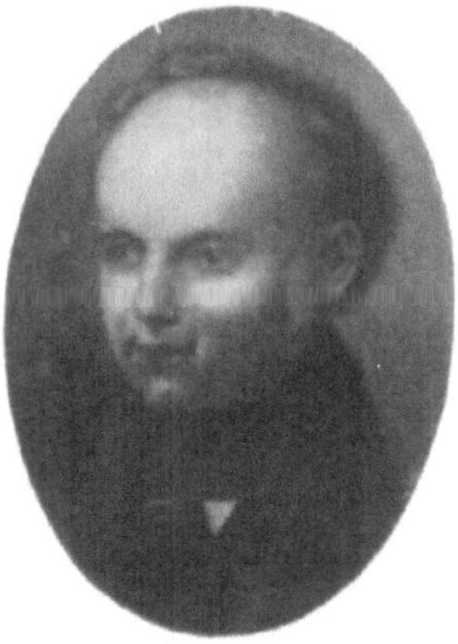

Mental Temperament

force, and he may lack that roughness and efficiency—necessary for struggle and competition—which makes the wide-headed man successful.

A *head very broad across the parietal eminences* is cautious, circumspect, given to inferiority and anxiety complexes; sensitive to impressions affecting the person, yet slow to anger and does not take the initiative readily.

A head with a *large occiput* indicates richness of affection; it exhibits tender feelings, attachment to family, friends, and home—a very social disposition. This type deals successfully with people, and should be placed in positions where these characteristics are of value. Female heads generally are longer than male heads at the back; and woman is more clinging in her love, and, speaking generally, more affectionate than man.

The larger occiput and strength of the tender emotion may account for the fact that women, when mentally ill, are more subject to melancholia; whilst men with their broader heads are better fitted for the roughness and struggles of life, and are more liable, in case of a mental breakdown, to suffer from acute mania.

Huschke and other observers have recorded their observation that the posterior lobes are more highly developed in women than in men, and, indeed, one rarely sees in women the straight back to the head so typical among men. It is not a question of coiffure, for one of the dominant distinctions of male and female skulls is this occipital development; moreover, it has been ascertained, by careful measurements, that women have more length of brain *posterior* to the fissure of Rolando than men, who correspondingly have more brain *anterior* to it. We must not forget, however, that there are women who are masculine in character and often in intelligence; and that there exist men with predominant female disposition.

HERMANN WELCKER found 73 per cent. of female skulls dolichocephalic (long-headed).

RICHTER (*Virchow's Archiv*, Vol. CXXVIII) and BROCA confirmed the results of Welcker. According to them it would appear that the greater length of the female head, as compared with that of the male, is due to the additional occipital length.

D. J. CUNNINGHAM, according to Havelock Ellis, assigned to women a longer occipital lobe. Dr. W. WEISBACH, in his book *Der deutsche Weiberschädel*, also testified to the larger occiput of women as compared with men.

CESARE LOMBROSO found in female criminals a short occiput; hence brachycephalic heads, and a complete absence of affection, though their libido sexualis was increased.

PAUL NÄCKE (*Archiv. f. Psychiatrie*, 1893), too, examined the brains of female criminals, and found that those committed for murder had deficient occipital lobes. In the others, thieves, etc., the occipital lobes were of normal size.

MORIZ BENEDIKT has described the brains of three murderesses, in whom the occipital lobes were short, and did not cover the cerebellum (*Verbrecher Gehirne*).

HERMANN MUNK said of a dog, the posterior lobes of which he had destroyed: "The sight of men, whom he used to greet joyfully, now leaves him cold, and even the company of dogs with whom he used to play leaves him unmoved"; thus showing loss of the gregarious instinct which gives social affection.

JACQUES LOEB found that after destruction of the most posterior part of the brain (occipital region) of a bitch, it lost its parental attachment, and neglected its puppies directly after delivery.

Monkeys, of all animals, are the first to possess distinct occipital convolutions covering the cerebellum; and they are considerably larger in the female than in the male, so that it is easy to distinguish the sexes by the appearance of their brains (see illustration). The female monkey, too, shows great, if not greater, attachment to its offspring than most animals, and orphan monkeys, according to BREHM, are always adopted and carefully guarded.

When anatomists set forth that the posterior lobes are entirely wanting in the lower animals—because the hemispheres of the brain do not extend backward far enough to overlap the cerebellum in the same way that they do in man—two factors have to be considered: (1) The circumstance of animal bodies being in the horizontal position, which demands such an accommodation as shall fit them for it; and (2) the difficulty of defining the anterior border line of the occipital lobe in the brains of animals.

All that is positively known about the functions of the occipital lobes is that the calcarine region is related to the sense of sight. This relationship was known to EMIL HUSCHKE, who wrote (*Schädel, Hirn, und Seele*, Jena, 1854):

"The posterior lobes, undoubtedly, are in ultimate relation with the emotional life and the sense of sight. No other sense organ has such an intimate connection with the tender feelings and grief as that of the nerve of sight, the fibres of which can be traced to the convolutions of the posterior lobes. Apart from the mimicry of the eye, in which all affections are most vividly reflected, weeping is the best of all proofs."

TAMBRONI (*Jahresbericht f. Neurologie u. Psychiatrie*) found in tumours of this region a disposition to weep.

G. ELLIOT SMITH (*British Medical Journal*, 1926: "We judge our fellow men and women by their movements, their gestures and expressions. We read their feelings and intentions in their facial movements, and feel that these speak a truer language than the words of articulate speech. In particular, *the eyes are the more eloquent signals of the sentiments and emotions*; a fact that finds ample expression, not merely in the common experience of every human being, but also in our common speech and poetry.

TEMPERAMENTS

The observation of heads, as an indication of ability and character, is not always so simple; for it has to be remembered that the brain is only the apparatus for the manifestation of intelligence. I have already mentioned that large frontal lobes are useless without a proper stock of information. It may be, also, that there is not the necessary character stimulus; that the person is easy-going, wanting in application, or deficient in nervous energy; or—what is not uncommon—that he is a mere dreamer.

Other factors that influence intellectual activity are the condition of the blood and circulation, the state of the bodily organs, the quality of the brain substance, and, last but not least, the activity of the glandular system; especially of the thyroid, or so-called monkey gland, which has a powerful influence in retarding or accelerating bodily and mental functions. Above all, the manifestation of intellectual and character dispositions is modified by the general temperament or constitution.

Thirty years ago, in 1901, I described three chief temperaments: (1) The vital; (2) the motive; and (3) the mental. These have now become popular under different names, invented by KRETSCHMER (*Physique and Character*, 1925); namely as (1) the pyknic; (2) the athletic; and (3) the asthenic. Kretschmer's book and theories have gained a high popularity in Germany; but his descriptions are in many respects similar to those I have given.

The *vital temperament* is characterised by a predominance of the internal organs of the body that generate life and help to sustain it, over the nervous system and bony and muscular frame. It is marked by a preponderance of the nutritive organs; the organs of digestion, respiration, and circulation, which occupy the greater cavities of the trunk. There is *fullness of the body, rotundity of the abdomen, plumpness and tapering limbs,* with hands and feet relatively small. The body is, generally, found *well covered with adipose tissue*; and persons of this temperament are known to be frank and good-natured.

Dr. Kretschmer calls this the "pyknic" type of build, which, he says, "as the name implies, is *short and fat. The limbs are well rounded*", and in the older members of this class there is often *pronounced fatness of the lower part of the trunk.*

Persons of the vital temperament, I indicated, must be ever doing something to work off their constantly accumulating stock of vitality; but they generally love play better than hard work. Their motto is: "*Let us live while we do live*". They are generally zealous, enthusiastic, impulsive; an enjoy the pleasures of animal life. For life's enjoyment there must be abundant vitality in the system. Such persons are interested in things present, and the subjects of everyday life. They are *warm, genial, placid,* contented, easy; fond of comfort and domesticity. They like to eat heartily; and like to have you eat heartily with them. *They are fond of a good story and a hearty laugh.*

The man of vital temperament, when in good health, is comfortable, physically. He does not suffer from the high nervous tension and physical frailty of the thinker. *Neither is he restless; but has poise,* ponders things, and has calm judgment. His comfort and good feeling make him genial and good-natured. Generally he is a man of heart, *who is happiest in his social relations,* a pleasant comrade, and a gay companion. *He makes acquaintances readily,* and imparts warmth and confidence to everyone around him. He attracts others, and gets them to do things for him. He supplies the wages, and profits by the efforts of the thinker and doer. The thinker searches for him for new facts, discoveries, inventions; the doer puts these into operation for him.

Kretschmer has a special name for these kind of people. He calls them "cyclothymes", meaning, "people who are *jolly, who take the world as it comes, whose emotions are easily roused and soon calmed, who are universally popular, and have a wide circle of acquaintances*".

The *motive temperament* is another variety of the human constitution, marked by a *superior development of the bony and muscular systems*. It embraces the bones and muscular framework. It is the machinery of the body.

The motive temperament does not give fineness to the texture of the body, or quality of the mind; but is distinguished *by broad shoulders, marked facial bones, large hands and large feet*, which are significant of utility rather than ornament. In this temperament the nutrition of the body seems to be drawn, chiefly, towards the maintenance of muscular action. *It imparts a delight in active exercise*, accompanied by endurance and toughness. Those who engage in bold enterprises—whose oratory is of the vehement and "sledge-hammer" kind—have this temperament.

Kretschmer called this kind of build the "athletic", and described it as "*broad-chested, heavily boned, with large extremities. The cheekbones are prominent, and the contour of the jaw is well marked.*"

Persons of this temperament have strength and endurance, unlimited capacity for hard work, particularly of a physical kind. They are generally slow-minded; not quick, but thorough. The facial expression is one of earnestness and determination. As a rule, they are distinguished for their force of character, industry, and executive ability; they have love of power, are the leaders in active life, observers rather than thinkers. Their success is by means of energy and perseverance; rather than through forethought, or deep scheming. They are men of the field; men with whom to think, and to feel, means to act. Their motto is: "*I work and I execute*". Persons who have this temperament are not so polished and refined in their manners as those who have the mental temperament, together with the same opportunities for mingling in refined society. They are more thorough, plodding, tenacious, plain, practical, efficient, and persevering. Pioneering work calls strongly to them. They evince marked interest in moving things—machinery, mining, railway building, and, indeed, in every kind of construction and manual labour. An inherent desire for physical activity makes them explorers, soldiers, athletes; and they excel in sports and games. Their sphere of action must be wide and high. Having great love of freedom, they care not for work involving ordered restraint. They are not office workers, and have little love for books or theoretical study.

The *mental temperament* embraces the brain and nervous system. In this variety of constitution, *the head is large, in proportion to the size of the body, and the frame is comparatively slight.* The *face is generally oval*, mobile, and expressive. The personality is seldom imposing, but may be graceful and elegant. *Such people have small muscles*, compact in quality; adapted to rapid action, rather than strength. The *frontal part of the brain is prominent.* Refinement and delicacy, in fact, are, in general, the features of the entire bodily structure.

Dr. Kretschmer calls this the "asthenic" build: "*tall, thin, and small boned.* The *extremities are small*, and delicate. *The face is oval*, and rather *broader at the forehead* than at the jaws."

The brain is the most active organ in persons of the mental temperament; consequently, pursuits are chosen that engage the mind rather than the body. The mental temperament develops sensation, emotion, thought, and feeling. It is the literary, poetic, and artistic temperament; and is well marked in the romantic, emotional, spiritual people, in the man fond of theories, and in the dreamer. Men with the mental temperament are poorly qualified to cope with the selfish business world; to do manual work; to endure hardships or the rough and tumble of life. They possess a quick display of feeling and a lively succession of thought. Their brain makes the body its servant, and, consequently, they exhaust it more readily. Their motto is: "*I think and I plan*".

Generally, the temperaments are more or less combined, two elements predominating over the third, in the same man; *vital-motive*, *vital-mental*, or *motive-mental* temperament.

The *vital-motive* or *motive-vital* temperament qualifies for the physical work of life. It is not of an intellectual trend, and it contributes but little taste for pursuits demanding study. There may exist good application; and, with a well-shaped brain, there will be practical talent, clear perception, and sound judgment. But it is in the out-of-door activities of the world that this combination proves most successful.

The *vital-mental* or *mental-vital* temperament is, for the most part, a happy organisation. It imparts many attractive qualities, especially to women; for with it coexist warm affections, kindness, amiability, grace, sprightliness; and usually much personal beauty. Men of this stamp, if educated, are fond of social festivities—make good orators, and possess wit and understanding.

The *motive-mental* or *mental-motive* temperament imparts a refining influence to the athletic build. One so constituted

PLATE XLV

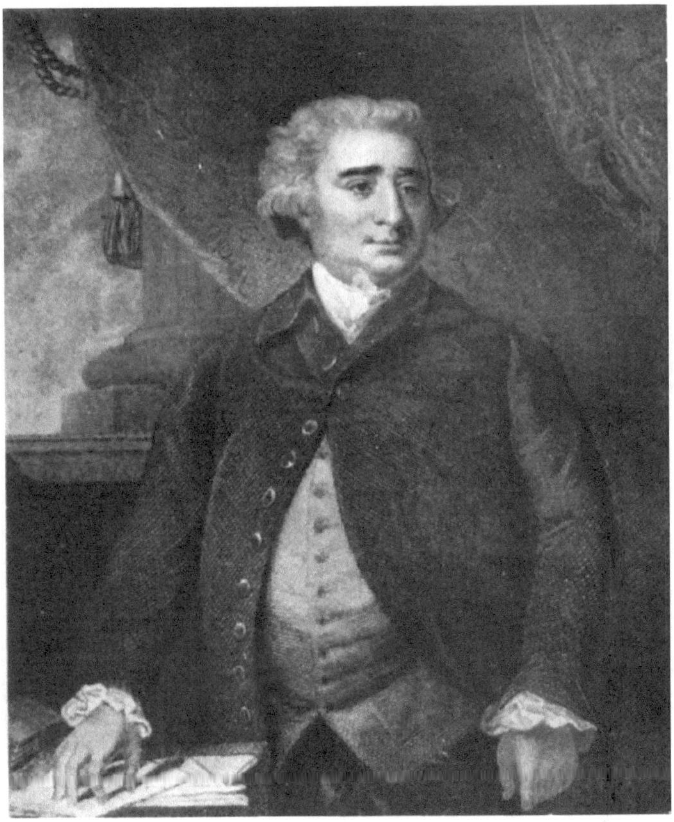

CHARLES JAMES FOX, STATESMAN

Vital temperament (*see page* 269)

PLATE XLVI

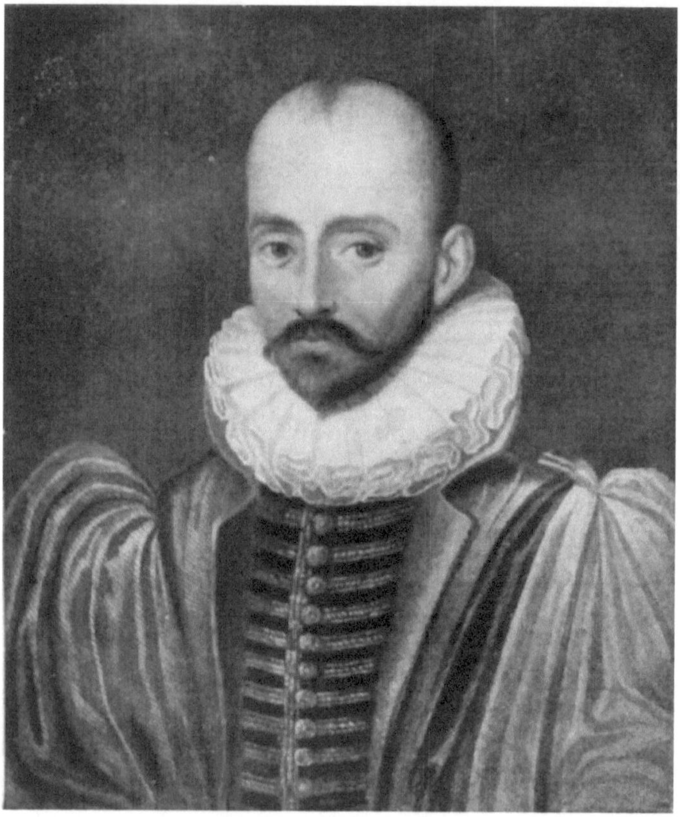

MONTAIGNE, PHILOSOPHER
Mental temperament (*see page* 271)

is clear-headed and energetic. He takes up solid, practical things; and is likely to take the lead. It implies a talent for planning, and power to carry out successfully. Those of this temperament are wishful to work, as well as to think; in fact, they think best while on their feet, carrying into effect their enterprises.

Conclusion

In conclusion, I should like to tender a further proof of the hypotheses advanced in this book: this is that the positions of the localisations—for the demonstration of which I have given so much evidence—are not accidental, but are governed by fixed principles. The localisations are of a higher character and of later acquisition, in proportion, as they occupy a higher locality in the brain. Thus the highest mental powers and of later acquisition—the ethical and aesthetical sentiments, etc.—are at the top of the head, in the superior part of the frontal convolutions, farthest from the base of the brain; for the rigid base of the skull does not admit of much extension. On the other hand, the lowest, and yet most indispensable, mental powers—the instincts of self-preservation, common to men and animals—will be found at the base of the brain, in the lower temporal and inferior parietal convolutions.

Further, it has been shown that the frontal lobes are destined for the intellectual processes, and the rest of the brain for the three primary emotions: the occipital lobes for love; the parietal, for fear; and the temporal lobes for anger.

Their morbid manifestations are similarly defined: the frontal lobes for the early stages of mania, and, later, for dementia; the parietal lobes for anxiety psychoses and melancholia; the temporal lobes for acute mania.

The vast collection of cases quoted in this volume serves to show:

(1) That lesions of the frontal lobes give rise to a feeling of joy, exaltation, and self-satisfaction, incessant enterprise, and a rapid flow of thought.

(2) That lesions of the parieto-occipital area give rise, generally, to low spirits, apprehensiveness, self-depreciation, depression, lack of initiative, slowness of ideas, and, often, a tendency to suicide.

(3) That lesions of the lower temporal area give rise to irritation, resentment, anger, aggressiveness, violence, and language in accordance with, and restricted to, these feelings, and often, also, to a tendency to epilepsy and homicide.

Postscript

Professor Constantin Economo, on March 20th, 1931, that is after this book was already in print, delivered a lecture before the Vienna Medical Association, in which he quite independently confirmed the main argument of the author. He said:

"The brain of man, though looking as if of uniform structure, consisted of anatomically differentiated areas, which must have distinctive functions. As a result of twenty years' research he had gained the conviction that not only had the human brain increased in size since ancestral times, but that it had increased in particular regions, which we may consider to be new acquisitions, indicating a progressive development concurrent with the intellectual growth of man. He was sure that *there must be an anatomical basis for the different innate human capacities and individual talents, and that not only does the brain still continue to develop, but it is quite possible that new 'organs' may be growing, giving man hitherto unsuspected abilities.*"

PLATE XLVII

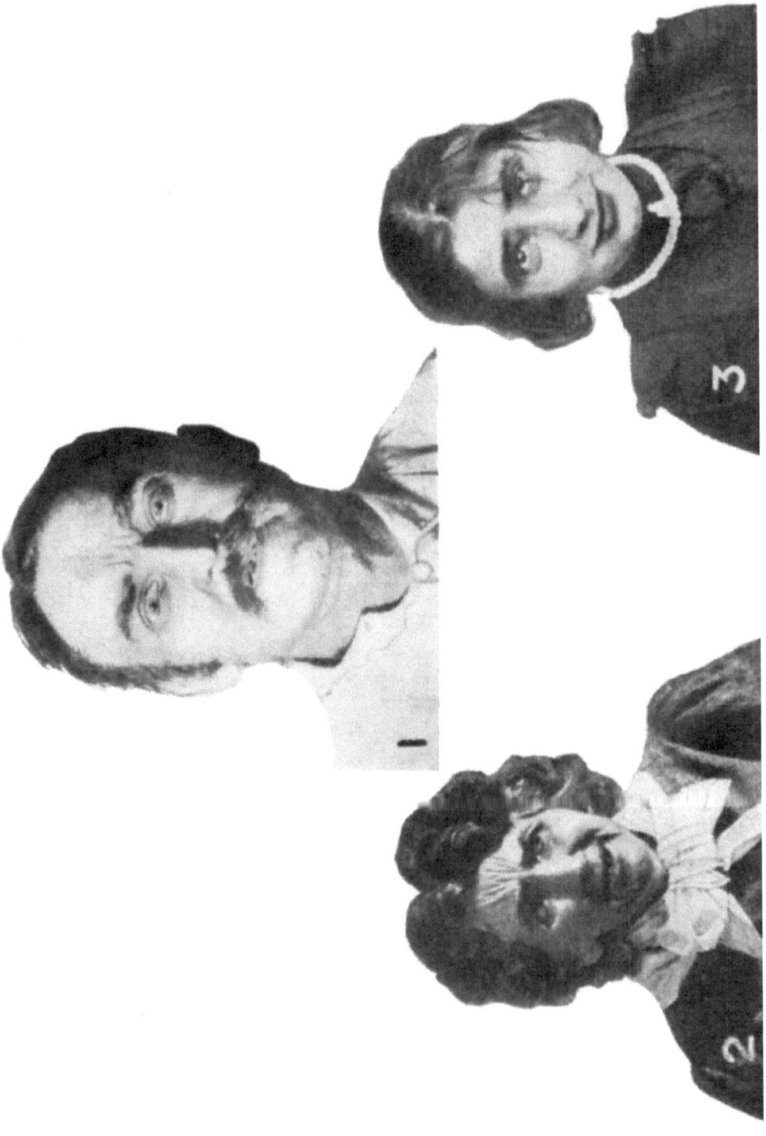

(1) PORTRAIT OF ANGRY, MANIACAL PATIENT (2) PORTRAIT OF ANXIOUS, MELANCHOLIC PATIENT
(3) PORTRAIT OF CHEERFUL, DEMENTED PATIENT

(*See page* 273)

LIST OF AUTHORS

SUBJECT INDEX